Study Guide to Accompany

Surgical Technology for the Surgical Technologist: A Positive Care Approach

The Association of Surgical Technologists, Inc.

Second Edition

Study Guide to Accompany

Surgical Technology for the Surgical Technologist: A Positive Care Approach

The Association of Surgical Technologists, Inc.

Second Edition

Teri L. Junge, CST/CFA
Surgical Technology Program Director
San Joaquin Valley College, Fresno, CA

THOMSON
DELMAR LEARNING™

Australia Canada Mexico Singapore Spain United Kingdom United States

THOMSON
DELMAR LEARNING™

Study Guide to Accompany Surgical Technology for the Surgical Technologist, Second Edition
The Association of Surgical Technologists
Teri L. Junge, CST/CFA

Vice President, Health Care Business Unit:
William Brottmilter

Editorial Director:
Cathy L. Esperti

Acquisitions Editor:
Rhonda Dearborn

Developmental Editor:
Marjorie A. Bruce

Marketing Director:
Jennifer McAvey

Marketing Coordinator:
Jill Osterhout

Editorial Assistant:
Natalie Wager

Art/Design Specialist:
Connie Lundberg-Watkins

Production Coordinator:
Bridget Lulay

Project Editor:
Jim Zayicek

Printed in the United States of America
5 XXX 08 07 06

For more information, contact Delmar Learning,
5 Maxwell Drive,
Clifton Park, NY 12065

or find us on the World Wide Web at
http://www.delmarlearning.com

Library of Congress Cataloging-in-Publication Data

ISBN 1-4018-3849-9

Contents

SKILL ASSESSMENT LIST AND LOCATOR

Skill Assessment (Name and Number)

Chapter 7

Asepsis and Sterile Technique

Chapter 8

General Patient Care and Safety

Chapter 9

Surgical Pharmacology and Anesthesia

Chapter 10

Instrumentation, Equipment, and Supplies

Chapter 11

Wound Healing, Sutures, Needles, and Stapling Devices

Chapter 12

Surgical Case Management

Preface

TO THE SURGICAL TECHNOLOGY STUDENT

The textbook ***Surgical Technology for the Surgical Technologist: A Positive Care Approach,*** second edition defines the cognitive model necessary for the surgical technologist to function effectively and provides an innovative approach for learning the role of the surgical technologist while focusing on the knowledge and skills that will be required. This model leads the way for the surgical technology student to remember the pertinent information using the predictive model: ***A Positive Care Approach.*** Because the text was written by surgical technologists and surgical technology educators, the needs of the student have been considered throughout the process. The graduate of a CAAHEP (Commission on Accreditation of Allied Health Education Programs) accredited surgical technology program will meet the eligibility requirements of the LCC-ST (Liaison Council on Certification for the Surgical Technologist) to sit for the national certifying examination for the surgical technologist.

The basic steps of the cognitive process for the surgical technologist are defined by Bob Caruthers, CST, PhD, former Deputy Director, Association of Surgical Technologists.

The surgical technologist:

- has a mental image of normal anatomy
- makes a mental comparison of the idealized anatomy with the actual anatomy of a specific patient
- knows an idealized operative procedure used to correct the pathologic condition
- makes a mental comparison of the idealized procedure with the actual procedure being performed
- allows for a particular surgeon's variations to the idealized procedure
- allows for variances in anatomy, pathology, and surgeons' responses to the variances
- predicts and prepares to meet the needs of the surgeon and surgical patient prior to verbalization of the need

To facilitate the learning process, *Surgical Technology for the Surgical Technologist: A Positive Care Approach* has been divided into two major sections. These divisions correspond to *A Positive Care Approach* and are represented by the A POSitive and CARE acronyms. The first 12 chapters are related to the CARE acronym. The CARE division itself is divided into two sections: (1) Introduction to Surgical Technology, and (2) Principles and Practice of Surgical Technology. The last 12 chapters relate to the A POSitive acronym; a brief introduction to diagnostics is followed by chapters focusing on operative procedures for various surgical specialties.

What is the *A Positive Care Approach?* It is a systematic approach to surgical problem solving focused on the ability of the surgical technologist to predict the needs of the surgeon and patient. The *A Positive Care Approach* uses two simple memory tools for systematic problem solving.

The CARE division will establish a broad context in which the instructor will help the student place the more specific technical information that dominates surgical technology. Introductory and foundational information is learned using the CARE approach, which is intended to serve as a reminder to the surgical technologist that all activities affect the care given to the patient. The student should be aware that the highly variable topics of the first 12, or non-procedural, chapters of the text do not allow a simple one-to-one correlation of the CARE memory tool, rather, it is a conceptual tool intended to help organize the information:

C Care directed toward the patient and/or surgical team

A Aseptic principles and practice of sterile technique

R Role of the surgical technologist

E Environmental awareness and concern

The A POSitive division relates directly to the final 12, or procedural, chapters with CARE as the underlying theme. The surgical procedures are presented by surgical specialty using the illustrative procedure format. The illustrative procedure format is based on the concept that one procedure can highlight several important steps that are repeated in related procedures. Rather than presenting many procedures with brief outlines of the steps, fewer procedures are presented in greater detail, thus allowing the surgical technologist to predict the necessary preparation and action to be taken. The A POSitive approach does allow the one-to-one correlation of the procedural chapter objectives and should be used to reinforce every surgical procedure encountered by the student:

A Anatomy

P Pathology

O Operative Procedure

S Specific Variations

In this Study Guide, we will provide you with learning concepts and tools and a way to use them to enhance your education.

The authors of ***Surgical Technology for the Surgical Technologist: A Positive Care Approach,*** second edition, wish you success in your endeavor to become a Certified Surgical Technologist (CST)!

CHAPTER 1

Orientation to Surgical Technology

OBJECTIVES

After studying this chapter, the reader should be able to:

C 1. Identify and demonstrate principles of communication in the surgical setting.

A 2. (No objectives focused on asepsis in this chapter; however, the student should demonstrate an awareness that the principles of asepsis are a vital component of the surgical technologist's role in surgical patient care.)

R 3. Trace the historical development of surgery and surgical technology.

4. Identify members of the surgical team and their roles.
5. Identify the various roles of the surgical technologist.
6. Identify and interpret a job description for the surgical technologist.

E 7. Identify different types of health care facilities.

8. Describe a typical hospital organizational structure.
9. Identify hospital departments and their relationship to surgical services.

Select Key Terms

Define the following:

1. acronym ______________________________
2. ambulatory surgical facility ______________________________
3. ARC-ST ______________________________
4. AST ______________________________
5. circulator ______________________________
6. competency ______________________________
7. Core Curriculum ______________________________
8. DO ______________________________
9. elective ______________________________
10. emergent ______________________________
11. HMO ______________________________
12. intraoperative ______________________________
13. JCAHO ______________________________
14. LCC-ST ______________________________
15. optional ______________________________
16. Pasteur ______________________________
17. postoperative ______________________________
18. preceptor ______________________________
19. preoperative ______________________________
20. professional ______________________________
21. proprietary ______________________________
22. STSR ______________________________
23. urgent ______________________________
24. Vesalius ______________________________

Case Studies

☐ CASE STUDY 1

Rodrigo is a 57-year-old male who was admitted to the emergency department (ED) following a motor vehicle accident. Rodrigo was driving a delivery van that was struck head-on by another vehicle. Rodrigo has severe injuries to both lower extremities: (1) closed femur fracture of the left leg and (2) open fracture of the right tibia and fibula with near amputation. A chest tube was inserted upon arrival in the ED. Rodrigo is neurologically intact. He is now scheduled for surgery on his legs.

1. This case represents what category of surgical intervention? ______________________________

2. What is the difference between emergent and urgent surgical intervention? ______________________________

3. What is elective surgery? ______________________________

4. Is elective surgical intervention the same thing as "minor" surgery? ______________________________

☐

☐ CASE STUDY 2

Kathleen is a 15-year-old female who has been admitted to the hospital for surgery to correct a condition called scoliosis, an abnormal lateral curvature of the spine. This surgical intervention requires a lengthy incision and dissection of spinal muscles. It runs the risk of considerable blood loss and damage to spinal nerves. Distraction rods are placed to help straighten the spine, and bone grafting is required.

1. Intraoperative X-rays are required. Who would perform these, and what department of the hospital would employ them? ______________________________

2. Blood loss may be countered by filtering the patient's blood and returning it to her. Who would perform this activity? ______________________________

3. Patients undergoing spinal surgery are often monitored for changes in electrical conduction to the lower extremities. Who would perform this task? ______________________________

4. To whom would blood samples be taken in order to check the hematocrit and hemoglobin counts during the operative procedure? ______________________________

5. An upper body cast may be applied several days postoperatively. Who would assist the surgeon in this task? ______________________________

☐

CHAPTER 2 Standards of Conduct

OBJECTIVES

After studying this chapter, the reader should be able to:

C 1. Analyze major concepts inherent in professional practice law.

2. Interpret the legal responsibilities of the surgical technologist and other surgical team members.

3. Analyze the American Hospital Association's Patient's Bill of Rights.

4. Describe the need for professional liability insurance policies.

A 5. Analyze the key elements related to developing a surgical conscience.

R 6. Assess the resources that aid the surgical technologist in interpreting and following professional standards of conduct.

7. Develop an increased sensitivity to the influence of ethics in professional practice.

8. Analyze the role of morality during ethical decision making.

9. Cite examples of ethical situations and problems in the health professions.

10. Analyze scope of practice issues as they relate to surgical technology.

11. Evaluate the role of the risk management department in the health care facility.

E 12. Apply principles of problem solving in ethical decision making.

13. Assess errors that may occur in the operating room and devise a plan for investigation, correction, and notification.

Select Key Terms

Define the following:

1. abandonment ______________________
2. accreditation ______________________
3. advance directive ______________________
4. affidavit ______________________
5. bioethics ______________________
6. clinical ladder program ______________________
7. code of ethics ______________________
8. credentialing ______________________
9. deontological approach ______________________
10. ethics ______________________
11. formalism ______________________
12. incident report ______________________
13. informed consent ______________________
14. job description ______________________
15. liability ______________________
16. malpractice ______________________
17. moral principles ______________________
18. negligence ______________________
19. Patient's Bill of Rights ______________________
20. risk management ______________________
21. Safe Medical Device Act ______________________
22. scope of practice ______________________
23. surgical conscience ______________________
24. tort law ______________________
25. utilitarianism ______________________

Case Studies

CASE STUDY 1

Mollie is a 9-year-old female admitted to the hospital following a seizure on the playground at school. She has been diagnosed with a cerebral arteriovenous malformation (AVM). A craniotomy with attendant clipping and removal of the AVM has been proposed. Mollie is in a foster home. Her biological parents are both dead.

1. What is needed for a valid consent for surgery in this case? ______________________

2. Who can give consent in this case? ______________________

3. Can the surgical intervention be refused? ______________________

☐ CASE STUDY 2

Harold is still a relatively new surgical technologist. Since passing the national certification examination, he has been working in a large teaching hospital. He loves the work and being at a hospital "on the cutting edge." He is surprised to find out that several of the staff members do not think they should be performing some of the procedures they do. They feel that it is experimenting on human beings.

1. Do you believe health care professionals are required to do everything necessary to save and prolong human life? ______________________________

2. What is more important: quality or quantity of life? How do you know what quality is? ______________________________

3. Is there such a thing as a "right to die"? ______________________________

4. Does a health care professional have the right to refuse to participate in approved procedures? ______________________________

☐

CHAPTER 3

The Surgical Patient

OBJECTIVES

After studying this chapter, the reader should be able to:

C 1. Assess the patient's response to illness and hospitalization.

A 2. Demonstrate awareness that all surgical patients have the right to the highest standards and practices in asepsis.

R 3. Distinguish and assess the physical, spiritual, and psychological needs of a patient.

E 4. Distinguish and assess cultural and religious influences on the surgical patient.

Select Key Terms

Define the following:

1. Maslow's hierarchy of needs ______________________________
2. patient ______________________________
3. physical need ______________________________
4. psychological need ______________________________
5. social need ______________________________
6. spiritual need ______________________________

Case Studies

CASE STUDY 1

Myrtle is scheduled for a total hip arthroplasty in about half an hour. She is in the preoperative holding area and has just expressed to her nurse a fear that she will not survive the procedure. Myrtle has asked to speak with the chaplain.

1. What type of need is Myrtle expressing? ______________________________
2. Should her premonition be taken seriously? ______________________________
3. With the procedure scheduled to take place shortly, will time allow the chaplain to be called? ______________________________

☐ CASE STUDY 2

The circulator has just come to the preoperative holding area to pick up 18-month-old Henry to take him to the operating room for his ear surgery. Henry took one look at the circulator and began screaming and clinging to his mother.

1. Use the life tasks approach to determine if Henry's behavior is appropriate for his age group. ______

2. Using Maslow's hierarchy of needs, which of Henry's needs may not be met when he is taken from his mother by the circulator to go to the operating room? ______

3. What can be done to make the transition from being in his mother's care to being in the care of the circulator a smooth one for Henry? ______

☐

CHAPTER 4

Special Populations

OBJECTIVES

After studying this chapter, the reader should be able to:

C 1. Compare and contrast the surgical care considerations for pediatric patients and patients who are obese, diabetic, pregnant, immunocompromised, disabled, geriatric, or experiencing trauma.

2. Describe the unique physical and psychological need of each special population.

A 3. Compare and contrast the intraoperative considerations for pediatric patients and patients who are obese, diabetic, immunocompromised, geriatric, or traumatized that relate to postoperative wound healing.

R 4. Evaluate the role of the surgical technologist for the surgical care of each special population.

E 5. Assess the ethical commitment that is required of surgical technologists as it relates to special populations care.

6. Describe the general needs associated with special populations of surgical patients.

Select Key Terms

Define the following:

1. arterial blood gases (ABGs) ______________________
2. autoimmune diseases ______________________
3. central venous catheter ______________________
4. diabetes mellitus ______________________
5. enterocolitis ______________________
6. golden hour ______________________
7. human immunodeficiency virus (HIV) ______________________
8. hypothermia ______________________
9. immunocompetence ______________________
10. intra-arterial measurement ______________________
11. Kaposi's sarcoma ______________________
12. kinematics ______________________
13. penetrating trauma ______________________
14. pneumothorax ______________________
15. Revised Trauma Score ______________________
16. septic shock ______________________
17. splenectomy ______________________
18. splenomegaly ______________________
19. torticollis ______________________
20. urine output ______________________
21. venous compression device ______________________

Case Studies

☐ CASE STUDY 1

Seven-year-old Alexandra lost control of her scooter as she was riding down her sloped driveway. She inadvertently rode into the street and was hit by a car. She was not wearing a helmet.

1. What is the first priority of the emergency team that arrives at the scene to assist Alexandra? ____________

2. The emergency team suspects that Alexandra may have sustained a neck injury during the accident. What should be done to protect the spinal cord? ____________

3. Alexandra appears to be going into hypovolemic shock. What step(s) should be taken to prevent the hypovolemia from becoming severe? ____________

☐

☐ CASE STUDY 2

Baby boy Daniels' birth was traumatic. He has suffered a bone fracture and the left side of his face appears to droop.

1. What is the most common type of bone fracture that occurs during traumatic birth?

2. What is most likely causing the neonate's face to droop?

3. Is the facial droop expected to resolve? If so, how soon?

CHAPTER 5

Physical Environment and Safety Standards

OBJECTIVES

After studying this chapter, the reader should be able to:

C 1. Identify and describe hazards to the patient in the operative environment.

2. Identify support services that work with the OR team in the care of the patient.

A 3. Understand the type of air-handling system required in the OR and the temperature and humidity required to maintain a sterile field.

4. Identify cleaning procedures, traffic patterns, and routines required in the operative environment.

R 5. Identify the role of the surgical technologist in the protection of self, patients, and others from hazards in the operative environment.

E 6. Identify the design types of the OR.

7. Identify hospital departments that relate to surgical services.

8. Understand the working environment of the OR.

9. Identify the physical components of the OR.

Select Key Terms

Define the following:

1. airborne bacteria ______________________________
2. back table ______________________________
3. decontamination room ______________________________
4. electrosurgical unit ______________________________
5. hamper ______________________________
6. high-efficiency particulate air (HEPA) filter ______________________________
7. hypothermia ______________________________
8. ionizing radiation ______________________________
9. laminar air flow ______________________________
10. Mayo stand ______________________________
11. methyl methacrylate (MMA) ______________________________
12. Occupational Safety and Health Administration (OSHA) ______________________________
13. pathology department ______________________________
14. perfusionist ______________________________
15. personal protective equipment (PPE) ______________________________
16. plume ______________________________
17. postanesthesia care unit (PACU) ______________________________
18. prophylaxis ______________________________
19. restricted area ______________________________
20. Standard Precautions ______________________________
21. suction outlet ______________________________
22. surgical site infection (SSI) ______________________________
23. triboelectrification ______________________________
24. Universal Precautions ______________________________

Case Studies

☐ CASE STUDY 1

Eloise is preparing to scrub for an open reduction internal fixation (ORIF) of a tibial plateau fracture. Intraoperative X-rays will be taken.

1. What special communications with other departments/personnel will be necessary prior to this procedure? ______

2. Will Eloise need to wear any personal protective equipment (PPE) for this procedure? ______

3. Will the patient require any safety equipment during the procedure? ______

4. The presence of an X-ray tech in the room presents a special situation. What responsibility does Eloise have during this time? ______

☐

☐ CASE STUDY 2

Today is Saturday; the staff in the operating room is limited. Marcus has been assigned to a femoropopliteal bypass surgery that could take six to eight hours. During the week, the OR staff can expect to be relieved for lunch, but today Marcus knows that is unlikely to happen.

1. What can Marcus do in advance to physically prepare himself for this lengthy procedure? ______________

____

____

____

____

2. Are there any tips that you can give Marcus to reduce the strain on his body while the case is in progress? _____

____

____

____

____

☐

CHAPTER 6

Biomedical Science

OBJECTIVES

After studying this chapter, the reader should be able to:

C
1. Identify basic components of a computer system.
2. Describe electrical safety precautions.
3. Define terms related to physics.
4. Describe the basic concepts of robotics.

A
5. (No objectives focused on asepsis in this chapter; however, the practice of sterile technique will be necessary when using related equipment in the OR.)

R
6. Perform basic word processing, Internet, and e-mail functions.
7. Apply computer knowledge to safe patient care.
8. Describe the geometrical concepts of robotics and the mechanisms of the robotic system.

E
9. Describe the basic principles of electricity and their application in the OR.
10. Apply the principles of robotics to safe patient care practices in the OR.
11. Apply the principles of physics to safe patient care practices in the OR.

Select Key Terms

Define the following:

1. active electrode ______
2. Cartesian coordinate geometry ______
3. central processing unit (CPU) ______
4. circuit ______
5. degrees of freedom ______
6. dispersive (inactive) electrode ______
7. electrons ______
8. font ______
9. free electrons ______
10. generator ______
11. ground wire ______
12. hydraulic pressure ______
13. inertia ______
14. infrared waves ______
15. insulator ______
16. load ______
17. mass ______
18. modem ______
19. monitor ______
20. mouse ______
21. neutrons ______
22. periodic table ______
23. plasma ______
24. power ______
25. pressure ______
26. protons ______
27. quarks ______
28. refraction ______
29. resistance ______
30. switch ______
31. volume ______

32. weight ______________________________

33. X-rays ______________________________

Case Studies

CASE STUDY 1

Norman is a surgical technologist who is circulating during a hip nailing. During the surgical procedure, the surgeon asks to see the patient's X-rays and blood test results since hepatitis B may be involved. Norman is going to use the computer in the operating room to send an e-mail requesting that the Radiology Department's unit secretary immediately bring over the patient's X-rays. He will send another e-mail to the laboratory technologist requesting that the blood test results be e-mailed to him in the OR.

1. Which icon will Norman use to create a new e-mail message? Where is the icon located and what does it look like? ______________________________

2. Norman wants to emphasize the patient's name and facility identification number. Briefly describe two ways to create emphasis using word processing functions. ______________________________

3. Norman wants to ensure that the individual at the surgery department control desk sees the e-mail (so that he or she will know which OR to deliver the X-rays to when they arrive), but that individual does not need to reply. What function would Norman use? ______________________________

(continues)

☐ CASE STUDY 1 (*continued*)

4. Norman recently visited the CDC website and noticed an update on hepatitis B. List three ways that he can find that site again.

☐ CASE STUDY 2

A female patient is brought to the operating room for a right oophorectomy. The surgeon is planning to use the AESOP robotic system to perform the surgical procedure. The STSR is responsible for setting up the robotic manipulator before the patient enters the OR.

1. On which side of the operating table should the manipulator be placed?

2. For optimal positioning of the endoscope, should the manipulator be placed at the head, midsection, or foot of the operating table?

3. When positioning the manipulator, what additional mechanism can be used to create more clearance between the elbow of the manipulator and the patient?

CHAPTER 7

Asepsis and Sterile Technique

OBJECTIVES

After studying this chapter, the reader should be able to:

C 1. Discuss the relationship between the principles of asepsis and practice of sterile technique and surgical patient care.

2. Define and discuss the concept of surgical conscience.

A 3. Discuss the principles of asepsis.

4. Define the terms related to asepsis.

5. Discuss the sterile practices related to the principles of asepsis.

6. Identify the principles and procedures related to disinfection and sterilization.

R 7. Demonstrate competency related to the practice of sterile technique.

8. Demonstrate competency in the procedures related to disinfection and sterilization.

E 9. Discuss the surgical environment and the application of the principles of asepsis to the environment.

Select Key Terms

Define the following:

1. asepsis
2. autoclave
3. bioburden
4. biological indicator
5. Bowie-Dick test
6. chelation
7. chemical indicator
8. colonization
9. contaminated
10. emulsification
11. endoscope
12. event-related sterility
13. flash sterilization
14. immersion
15. integrity
16. intermediate-level disinfection
17. Julian date
18. Lister
19. lumen
20. pathogen
21. permeability
22. sterile field
23. sterile technique
24. sterilization
25. surgical conscience
26. ultrasonic washer

Case Studies

☐ CASE STUDY 1

Brittney telephones her physician to report that she is experiencing a fever of 101°F seven days following her laparoscopic tubal ligation. She also states that she is experiencing urinary frequency and burning during urination. The physician suspects that Brittney may be suffering from a urinary tract infection because of the catheter that was used to empty her bladder during the surgical procedure. The physician has asked Brittney to schedule an appointment later in the day so that he may examine her and obtain a "clean catch" urine sample.

1. Would Brittney's infection be considered a surgical site infection (SSI)? If not, what type of infection is it?

____

____

____

____

2. What is the most likely reason that Brittney is suffering from an infection?

____

____

____

____

☐

☐ CASE STUDY 2

Ned is preparing the operating room for an emergency procedure. He is rushing because he knows that the patient will soon be brought into the room and he may not have time to complete his preparations. Ned is opening the final item; just as he is about to place the item on the back table, he notices a small hole in the wrapper.

1. What moral/ethical concept will Ned use to make the "right" decision?

____

____

____

____

(continues)

☐ CASE STUDY 2 (*continued*)

2. What are Ned's options, and what is the best choice?

3. If Ned makes the wrong choice, what possible impact could this have on the patient?

Skill Assessment 7-1

Basic Handwash

Student Name ______________________ Date ______________

Instructor ______________________

Procedural Step	Adequate	Needs Review
1. Student is able to state purpose of handwash		
2. Student is able to state circumstances when a handwash is necessary		
3. Equipment and supplies are assembled		
4. Jewelry removed		
5. Turn on faucet		
6. Inspect hands and wrists		
7. Wet hands and wrists		
8. Apply soap		
9. Lather		
10. Interlace fingers		
11. Use nail cleaner/brush (if necessary)		
12. Handwash is of appropriate duration		
13. All surfaces cleaned		
14. Rinse		
15. Turn off water		
16. Dry		
17. Discard towel(s)		

Comments ______________________

Skill Assessment 7-2

Packaging Technique – Wrap (Envelope Fold)

Student Name ______________________ Date ____________

Instructor ______________________

Procedural Step	Adequate	Needs Review
1. Student is able to state purpose for envelope-style wrap		
2. Appropriate attire		
3. Wash hands (Standard Precautions)		
4. Equipment and supplies assembled		
5. Orient wrap material on suitable surface		
6. Place item to be wrapped on wrapper		
7. Insert internal indicator		
8. Fold first flap		
9. Fold second (left) flap		
10. Fold third (right) flap		
11. Fold fourth flap		
12. Apply second wrapper (if necessary)		
13. Secure final flap		
14. Label for processing		
15. Place in designated area		
16. Proceed with other tasks		

Comments ______________________

Skill Assessment 7-3

Packaging Technique – Wrap (Square Fold)

Student Name ______________________ Date ____________

Instructor ______________________

Procedural Step	Adequate	Needs Review
1. Student is able to state purpose for square-style wrap		
2. Appropriate attire		
3. Wash hands (Standard Precautions)		
4. Equipment and supplies assembled		
5. Orient wrap material on suitable surface		
6. Place item to be wrapped on wrapper		
7. Insert internal indicator		
8. Fold first flap		
9. Fold second flap		
10. Fold third flap		
11. Fold final flap		
12. Apply second wrapper (if necessary)		
13. Secure final flap		
14. Label for processing		
15. Place in designated area		
16. Proceed with other tasks		

Comments ______________________

Skill Assessment 7-4

Packaging Technique – Peel Pack

Student Name ______________________________ Date ______________

Instructor ______________________________

Procedural Step	Adequate	Needs Review
1. Student is able to state purpose for peel pack-style package		
2. Appropriate attire		
3. Wash hands (Standard Precautions)		
4. Equipment and supplies assembled		
5. Place item(s) in pouch		
6. Seal pouch		
7. Double package (if necessary)		
8. Label for processing		
9. Place in designated area		
10. Proceed with other tasks		

Comments ______________________________

____

____

____

Skill Assessment 7-5

Packaging Technique – Container System

Student Name ______________________________ Date ______________

Instructor ______________________________

Procedural Step	Adequate	Needs Review
1. Student is able to state purpose for container-style package		
2. Appropriate attire		
3. Wash hands (Standard Precautions)		
4. Equipment and supplies assembled		
5. Prepare container		
6. Place instrument set in basket		
7. Place basket in container		
8. Place lid and seal		
9. Label for processing		
10. Place in designated area		
11. Proceed with other tasks		

Comments ______________________________

____

____

____

CHAPTER 8

General Patient Care and Safety

OBJECTIVES

After studying this chapter, the reader should be able to:

C 1. Demonstrate an understanding of the process used to obtain an informed consent for a surgical procedure or treatment.

2. Describe preoperative routines.
3. Identify, describe, and demonstrate the principles of transportation of the surgical patient.
4. Discuss, demonstrate, and apply the principles of surgical positioning.
5. Understand the methods of preparation of the operative site for surgery.
6. Describe the application of thermoregulatory devices.
7. Explain the principles and demonstrate the taking and recording of vital signs.
8. Explain the principles of urinary catheterization and demonstrate the procedure.

A 9. Describe how the principles of operative site preparation and urinary catheterization are related both to patient care and to the principles of asepsis.

R 10. Discuss methods of hemostasis and blood replacement and demonstrate the preparation and use of appropriate agents or devices.

11. Identify developing emergency situations, initiate appropriate action, and assist in treatment of the patient.
12. Discuss methods and types of documentation used in the OR.

E 13. Discuss the relationship between patient safety and the surgical environment.

Select Key Terms

Define the following:

1. apical pulse ______________________________
2. autologous ______________________________
3. cardiac dysrhythmia ______________________________
4. catheterization ______________________________
5. CPR ______________________________
6. dyspnea ______________________________
7. hemolysis ______________________________
8. hemostasis ______________________________
9. hemostat ______________________________
10. homologous ______________________________
11. informed consent ______________________________
12. laser ______________________________
13. NPO ______________________________
14. prep ______________________________
15. prone ______________________________
16. pulse oximeter ______________________________
17. Rh factor ______________________________
18. sedation ______________________________
19. shock ______________________________
20. suction ______________________________
21. supine ______________________________
22. tourniquet ______________________________
23. vital signs ______________________________

Case Studies

☐ CASE STUDY 1

Viorel is a 10-year-old male who has been adopted. He is scheduled for a right inguinal herniorrhaphy.

1. Who has the authority to sign Viorel's operative consent?

2. In what position will Viorel be placed for the herniorrhaphy?

3. Describe the anatomical area that will be prepped.

4. Are any special considerations necesssary to accommodate Viorel's age?

☐ CASE STUDY 2

After Virginia-May was placed on the operating table, it was discovered that her surgeon would be delayed by approximately 15 minutes. Virginia-May is 67 years old and is scheduled for a vaginal hysterectomy. She is very apprehensive.

1. What steps can be taken to help Virginia-May feel more comfortable?

2. Should the operating team continue with the preparations? For example, should she be anesthetized and positioned?

☐

Skill Assessment 8-1

Vital Signs – Temperature

Student Name ______________________ Date ____________

Instructor ______________________

Procedural Step	Adequate	Needs Review
1. Student is able to state purpose for temperature monitoring		
2. Wash hands (Standard Precautions)		
3. Equipment and supplies are assembled		
4. Equipment prepared		
5. Identify patient, self, and explain procedure (if applicable)		
6. Position patient (if necessary)		
7. Place temperature probe		
8. Probe remains in position for prescribed amount of time		
9. Hold temperature probe in place (if necessary)		
10. Carefully remove temperature probe		
11. Read thermometer		
12. Wash hands (Standard Precautions)		
13. Record or report findings		
14. Care for equipment as needed		

Comments ______________________

Skill Assessment 8-2

Vital Signs – Pulse

Student Name ______________________________ Date ______________

Instructor ______________________________

Procedural Step	Adequate	Needs Review
1. Student is able to state purpose for pulse measurement		
2. Wash hands (Standard Precautions)		
3. Equipment and supplies are assembled		
4. Identify patient, self, and explain procedure (if applicable)		
5. Position patient (if necessary)		
6. Locate site		
7. Compress artery (or listen with stethoscope)		
8. Note time		
9. Count pulse rate and note rhythm, volume, and condition of the arterial wall		
10. Wash hands (Standard Precautions)		
11. Record or report findings		
12. Care for equipment as needed		

Comments ______________________________

____

____

____

Skill Assessment 8-3

Vital Signs – Respiration

Student Name ______________________________ Date ______________

Instructor ____

Procedural Step	Adequate	Needs Review
1. Student is able to state purpose of respiration monitoring		
2. Student is able to state normal respiration values, identify an abnormality, and explain the implications of an abnormality		
3. Wash hands (Standard Precautions)		
4. Equipment and supplies are assembled		
5. Identify patient, self, and explain procedure (if applicable)		
6. Position patient (if necessary)		
7. Obtain respiratory rate, depth, rhythm, and breath sounds		
8. Wash hands (Standard Precautions, if necessary)		
9. Record or report findings		
10. Care for equipment as needed		

Comments ____

____

____

____

Skill Assessment 8-4

Vital Signs – Blood Pressure

Student Name ______________________________ Date ______________

Instructor ____

Procedural Step	Adequate	Needs Review
1. Student is able to state purpose for blood pressure monitoring		
2. Student is able to state normal blood pressure values, identify an abnormality, and explain the implications of an abnormality		
3. Wash hands (Standard Precautions)		
4. Equipment and supplies are assembled		
5. Identify patient, self, and explain procedure (if applicable)		
6. Position patient and expose site (if necessary)		
7. Apply blood pressure cuff		
8. Place stethoscope		
9. Inflate blood pressure cuff		
10. Deflate blood pressure cuff slowly, while listening for Korotkoff's sounds		
11. Continue deflation of blood pressure cuff. Continue to note sounds		
12. Complete deflation of cuff and remove cuff (if situation allows)		
13. Wash hands (Standard Precautions)		
14. Record or report findings		
15. Care for equipment as needed		

Comments ____

____

____

____

Skill Assessment 8-5

Glove Oneself – Open Glove Technique (Not Recommended When Wearing a Sterile Gown)

Student Name ______________________________ Date ______________

Instructor ____

Procedural Step	Adequate	Needs Review
1. Student is able to state purpose for application of sterile gloves		
2. Student is able to give several examples of situations in which the open glove technique will be necessary		
3. Wash hands (Standard Precautions)		
4. Equipment and supplies are assembled		
5. Remove outer wrapper		
6. Open inner wrapper		
7. Secure first glove from wrapper		
8. Apply first glove		
9. Secure second glove from wrapper		
10. Apply second glove		
11. Keep gloved hands sterile		

Comments ____

Skill Assessment 8-6

Remove Soiled Gloves

Student Name ______________________________ Date ______________

Instructor ______________________________

Procedural Step	Adequate	Needs Review
1. Student is able to state purpose for using correct glove removal technique		
2. Student is able to give examples of several situations in which this technique will be employed		
3. Equipment and supplies are assembled		
4. Grasp palm of glove to be removed first with opposite hand		
5. Remove first glove		
6. Keep removed glove in hand that remains gloved		
7. Begin to remove second glove		
8. Contain first glove inside of inverted second glove		
9. Finish removal of second glove		
10. Properly dispose of gloves		
11. Wash hands (Standard Precautions)		

Comments ______________________________

____

____

____

Skill Assessment 8-7

Urinary Catheterization (Male or Female)

Student Name ______________________________ Date ______________

Instructor ______________________________

Procedural Step	Adequate	Needs Review
1. Student is able to define urinary catheterization		
2. Student is able to state purpose for urinary catheterization		
3. Student is able to identify several situations in which urinary catheterization will be needed		
4. Student is able to identify different types of equipment that may be needed and state examples of when each may be used		
5. Wash hands (Standard Precautions)		
6. Equipment and supplies are assembled		
7. Identify patient, self, and explain procedure (if applicable)		
8. Position and expose patient		
9. Provide adequate lighting		
10. Remove protective cover and open catheter kit		
11. Don sterile gloves		
12. Organize supplies within sterile field		
13. Apply sterile drapes		
14. Cleanse meatus		
15. Insert catheter		
16. Inflate balloon		
17. Position catheter		
18. Care for patient and supplies as needed		
19. Wash hands (Standard Precautions)		
20. Document procedure		

Comments ______________________________

Skill Assessment 8-8

Skin Prep

Student Name ______________________ Date ______________

Instructor ______________________

Procedural Step	Adequate	Needs Review
1. Student is able to define surgical skin prep		
2. Student is able to state purpose for surgical skin prep		
3. Student is able to identify several situations that will require skin prep		
4. Student is able to identify different types of equipment and supplies that may be needed		
5. Wash hands (Standard Precautions)		
6. Equipment and supplies are assembled		
7. Identify patient, self, and explain procedure (if applicable)		
8. Position and expose patient		
9. Provide adequate lighting		
10. Open prep set		
11. Don sterile gloves		
12. Organize supplies within sterile field		
13. Apply sterile drapes		
14. Apply antiseptic solution to patient's skin		
15. Dry		
16. Apply "paint"		
17. Care for patient and supplies as needed		
18. Wash hands (Standard Precautions)		
19. Document procedure		

Comments ______________________

CHAPTER 9

Surgical Pharmacology and Anesthesia

OBJECTIVES

After studying this chapter, the reader should be able to:

C

1. Define general terminology and abbreviations associated with pharmacology and anesthesia.
2. Describe the action, uses, and modes of administration of drugs and anesthetic agents used in the care of the surgical patient.
3. Describe the side effects and contraindications for use of drugs and anesthetic agents.
4. Describe the factors that influence anesthesia selection for individual patients.

A

5. Demonstrate safe practice in transferring drugs and solutions from the nonsterile area to the sterile field.
6. Demonstrate the procedure for identifying a drug or solution on the sterile field.
7. Explain how sterile technique is used in relation to certain anesthesia procedures.

R

8. Convert equivalents from one system to another and accurately identify, mix, and measure drugs for patient use.
9. Explain the roles of the STSR and circulator during the administration of anesthesia.

E

10. Discuss care and precautions in identifying drugs and solutions in the OR.
11. List the equipment used as an adjunct to anesthesia.

Select Key Terms

Define the following:

1. agonist ______
2. amnesia ______
3. anaphylaxis ______
4. anesthesia ______
5. antagonist ______
6. antimuscarinic ______
7. aspiration ______
8. biotechnology ______
9. buccal ______
10. capnography ______
11. contraindication ______
12. doppler ______
13. drug ______
14. generic ______
15. homeostasis ______
16. hypnosis ______
17. iatrogenic ______
18. indication ______
19. induction ______
20. intra-articular ______
21. laryngospasm ______
22. NPO ______
23. PACU ______
24. parenteral ______
25. pharmacodynamics ______
26. pharmacokinetics ______
27. pharmacology ______
28. prophylaxis ______
29. topical ______
30. volatile agents ______

Exercise A – Start and Maintain a Medication File

The student will keep an ongoing file of medications commonly used showing: Name of Drug—Generic Name (Trade Name), Drug Classification, Kinetics (drug action), Route(s) of Administration, Possible Iatrogenic, Adverse, or Idiosyncratic Reactions and Contraindications. (Index cards work well for this exercise.)

Additionally, the instructor may have the student include on the back of the card: Usual Dosages, Special Administration and Storage Instructions, Antagonist, Drug Interactions, Overdose Symptoms and Management, Preoperative Instructions, Pain Management, and Typical Onset, Peak Effect, and Duration Times.

Sample:

front

Drug Name: **Drug Classification:**

Drug Action: **Route(s) of Administration:**

Possible Iatrogenic, Adverse, or Idiosyncratic Reactions:

Contraindications:

back

Antagonist: **Special Administration and Storage Instructions:**

Usual Dosages: **Onset:**

Peak Effect:

Preoperatively:

Duration Time:

Pain Management:

Drug Interactions:

MAO Inhibitors:

Overdose Symptoms:

Overdose Management:

Exercise B – Metric Conversions

Perform the following computations and exercises. Refer to Table 9-3 in the textbook if necessary.

1. Identify the following abbreviations.

   A. C ________________

   B. m ________________

   C. kg ________________

   D. L ________________

   E. µL ________________

   F. F ________________

   G. mm ________________

   H. mg ________________

   I. g ________________

   J. dL ________________

   K. m ________________

   L. µg ________________

   M. mL ________________

   N. cm ________________

   O. km ________________

   P. cc ________________

2. Calculate the following weight conversions.

   A. 14 lb = ________________ kg

   B. 123 lb = ________________ kg

   C. 46 kg = ________________ lb

   D. 78 kg = ________________ lb

   E. 4000 g = ________________ kg

   F. 4000 g = ________________ lb

   G. 1 g = ________________ mg

   H. 2000 mg = ________________ oz

   I. 4 oz = ________________ g

   J. 114 g = ________________ mg

3. Calculate the following length conversions.

   A. 1 km = ________________ m

   B. 1000 m = ________________ miles

   C. 4 miles = ________________ km

   D. 2 m = ________________ inches

   E. 17 inches = ________________ cm

   F. 30 mm = ________________ inches

   G. 100 cm = ________________ inches

   H. 1 inch = ________________ cm

   I. 1 inch = ________________ mm

   J. 1 yard = ________________ cm

4. Calculate the following volume conversions.

   A. 1 mL = ________________ cc

   B. 4 cc = ________________ mL

   C. 2 oz = ________________ cc

   D. 5 liters = ________________ cc

   E. 1 dL = ________________ mL

   F. 0.102 oz = ________________ mL

   G. 500 cc = ________________ L

   H. 0.75 L = ________________ cc

   I. 0.034 oz = ________________ cc

   J. 12 mL = ________________ oz

5. Calculate the following temperature conversions.

   A. 4°C = ________________ F

   B. 32°F = ________________ C

   C. 98.6°F = ________________ C

   D. 0°F = ________________ C

   E. 18°C = ________________ F

   F. 101°F = ________________ C

   G. 104°F = ________________ C

   H. 212°F = ________________ C

   I. 81°C = ________________ F

   J. 91.4°F = ________________ C

Exercise C – Identification

1. The trade names for several commonly used medications are listed. Provide the generic name.

   A. Ancef ____________________

   B. Anectine ____________________

   C. Coumadin ____________________

   D. Dantrium ____________________

   E. Decadron ____________________

   F. Demerol ____________________

   G. Forane ____________________

   H. Gelfoam ____________________

   I. Humulin ____________________

   J. Kantrex ____________________

   K. Lasix ____________________

   L. Marcaine ____________________

   M. Miochol ____________________

   N. Narcan ____________________

   O. Pitocin ____________________

   P. Robinul ____________________

   Q. Sublimaze ____________________

   R. Tagamet ____________________

   S. Toradol ____________________

   T. Tracrium ____________________

   U. Tylenol ____________________

   V. Valium ____________________

   W. Versed ____________________

   X. Wydase ____________________

2. Identify the components of the syringe shown in Figure 9-1.

   A. ____________ D. ____________

   B. ____________ E. ____________

   C. ____________

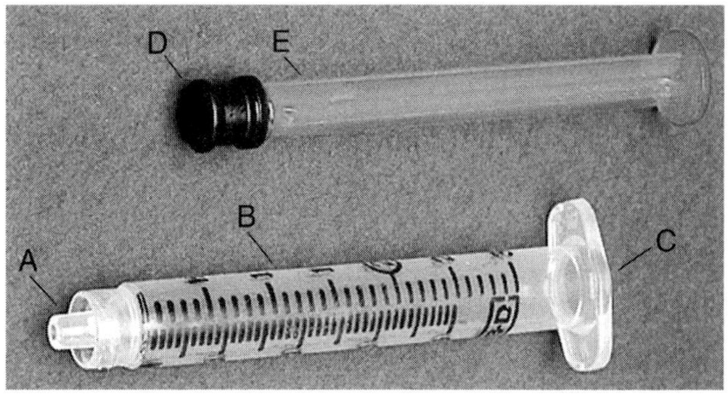

Figure 9-1

3. Identify the components of the needle shown in Figure 9-2.

   A. ____________ D. ____________

   B. ____________ E. ____________

   C. ____________ F ____________

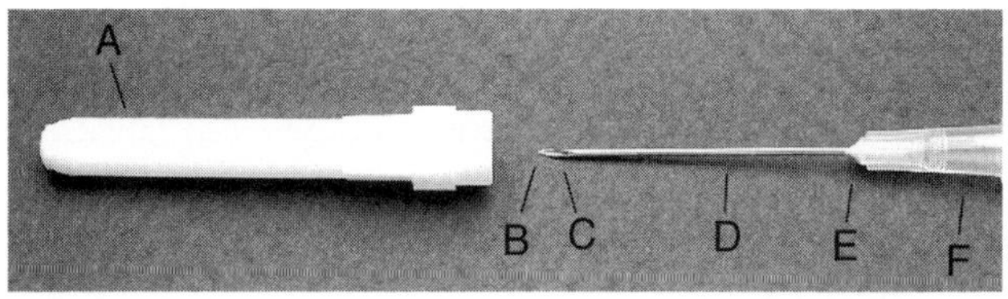

Figure 9-2

4. The physician has ordered 5,000 units of heparin. What volume of heparin will be needed? Use the medication labels pictured in Figure 9-3 to determine your answer. ____________________

   ____

   ____

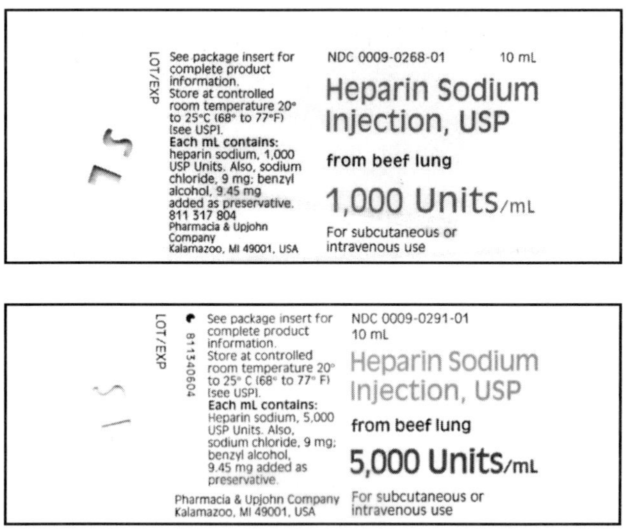

Figure 9-3 (Courtesy of the Upjohn Company)

5. From which source is heparin derived? ____________

____

6. The surgeon preference card calls for topical thrombin. Where will the STSR initially locate the medication? ____________

____

7. In which drug form is topical thrombin manufactured? ____________

____

8. What must be done to prepare the medication for use? ____________

____

9. What unit of measure is used to determine the dosage of topical thrombin? Use the medication label pictured in Figure 9-4 to determine your answer. ____________

____

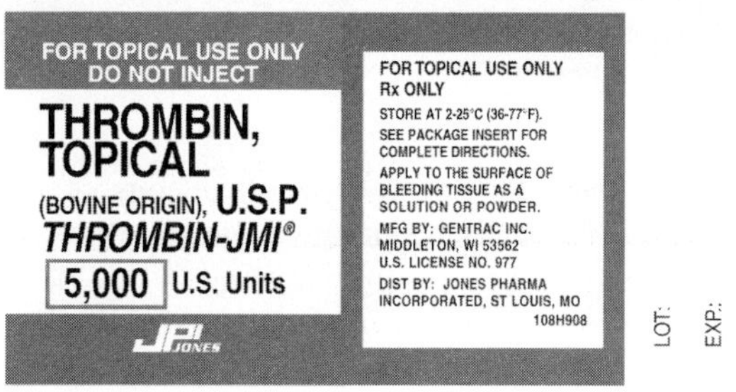

Figure 9-4 (Courtesy of Jones Pharma)

10. The physician has ordered 100,000 units of bacitracin, diluted in 1,000 cc of saline, for irrigation of the abdominal cavity. How many vials of bacitracin will be needed? Use the medication label pictured in Figure 9-5 to determine your answer. ____________

____

11. In which drug form is bacitracin manufactured?

____

12. What must be done to prepare bacitracin for use? ____________

____

13. How will the bacitracin/saline solution be introduced into the abdominal cavity? What supplies will be necessary? ____________

____

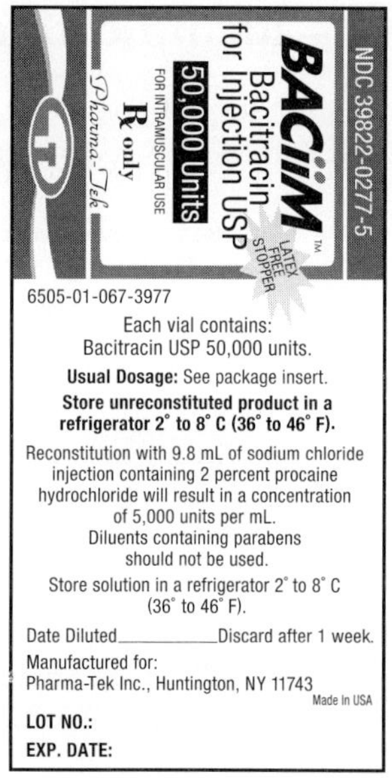

Figure 9-5 (Courtesy of Pharma-Tek, Inc.)

14. Cocaine HCl 4% has been ordered as a local anesthetic for a patient having nasal surgery. Will the cocaine be injected? ____________

____

15. What is the drug classification for cocaine? ____________

____

16. If any cocaine remains at the end of the procedure, is any special procedure necessary to ensure proper disposal? Why? ____________

____

17. The physician preference card calls for 1 g of kanamycin. How many vials of kanamycin will be needed? Use the medication label in Figure 9-6 to determine your answer. ____________

____

18. What is the drug classification for kanamycin?

____

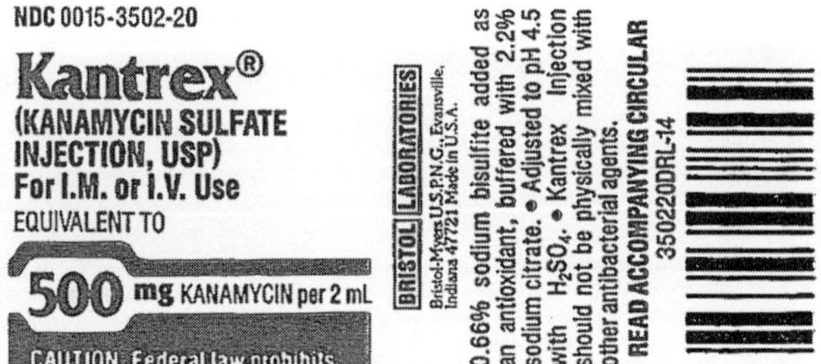
NDC 0015-3502-20
Kantrex®
(KANAMYCIN SULFATE INJECTION, USP)
For I.M. or I.V. Use
EQUIVALENT TO
500 mg KANAMYCIN per 2 mL
CAUTION: Federal law prohibits dispensing without prescription.
BRISTOL LABORATORIES
Bristol-Myers U.S.P.N.C., Evansville, Indiana 47721 Made in U.S.A.
0.66% sodium bisulfite added as an antioxidant, buffered with 2.2% sodium citrate. • Adjusted to pH 4.5 with H2SO4. • Kantrex Injection should not be physically mixed with other antibacterial agents.
READ ACCOMPANYING CIRCULAR
350220DRL-14
MAXIMUM DAILY DOSE: 1.5 GRAM

Figure 9-6 (Courtesy of Apothecon)

19. For what purpose would kanamycin be ordered?

____

20. What is the drug classification for oxytocin?

____

21. In what situation(s) in the operating room is the use of oxytocin indicated? ____________________

____

22. The surgeon has requested that the STSR have 20 units of oxytocin available on the sterile field. How many vials will be necessary? Use the medication label in Figure 9-7 to determine your answer. ______

____

23. Via which route(s) is oxytocin administered?

____

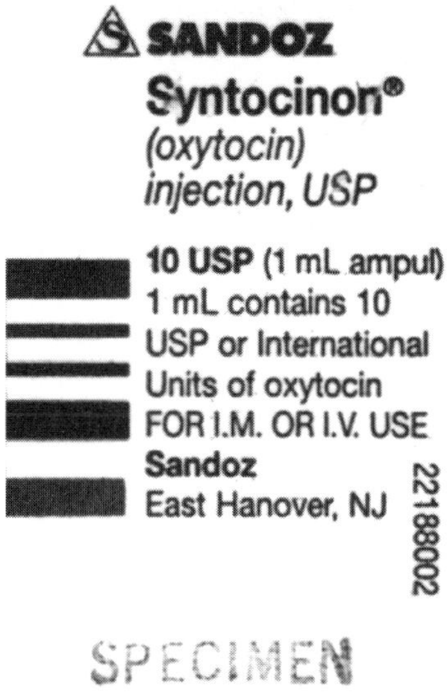

Figure 9-7 (Courtesy of Novartis Pharmaceuticals Corp.)

Case Studies

☐ CASE STUDY 1

Amanda, a 22-month-old female, is scheduled to have a percutaneous liver biopsy under general anesthesia at 7:30 AM. Her mother states that she has been NPO since last evening when she drank a bottle of 2% milk about 8:00 PM.

1. Why will Amanda be having a general anesthetic?

____

____

____

____

2. Has Amanda been NPO for an adequate amount of time?

____

____

____

____

(continues)

☐ CASE STUDY 1 (*continued*)

3. How will the anesthetist determine the approximate size of Amanda's trachea?

4. How are pediatric drug dosages calculated?

5. What special anesthesia equipment, if any, will be needed to care for Amanda?

☐

☐ CASE STUDY 2

Tony, an 86-year-old male, is scheduled for a ventral herniorrhaphy with general anesthesia. An IV line has been inserted in Tony's left forearm. You have been asked to assist the anesthesiologist and the circulator as they position Tony on the operating table and apply the devices that will be used to monitor his condition while he is anesthetized.

1. Will Tony's position remain the same for his anesthetic administration and the procedure? What position(s) will be necessary?

☐ CASE STUDY 2 (*continued*)

2. Place the following monitors and safety devices on Tony. Indicate placement by writing the corresponding letters on the diagram of Tony (Figure 9-8). Provide your rationale for each placement decision.

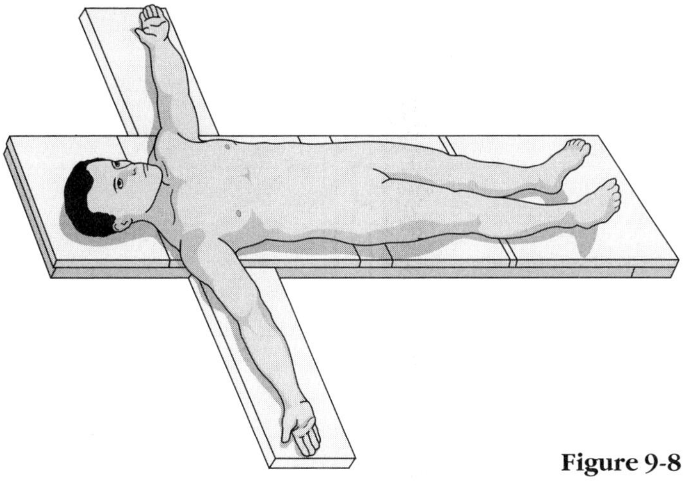

Figure 9-8

A. IV— ______________________________

____

B. Thermometer— ______________________________

____

C. Blood Pressure Cuff— ______________________________

____

D. Pulse Oximeter— ______________________________

____

E. Safety Strap— ______________________________

____

F. Electrosurgical Grounding Pad— ______________________________

____

G. 5-Lead ECG Electrodes— ______________________________

____

3. Show the area that will be prepped by lightly shading it in on Tony's figure. Why is it important to consider the skin prep when placing monitors?

____

____

____

☐

Skill Assessment 9-1

Sellick's Maneuver

Student Name ______________________ Date ______________

Instructor ______________________

Procedural Step	Adequate	Needs Review
1. Student is able to define Sellick's Maneuver		
2. Verbalize purpose of Sellick's Maneuver		
3. Give two examples in which Sellick's Maneuver may be indicated		
4. Position self properly		
5. Identify relevant anatomy		
6. Position hand properly		
7. Apply adequate pressure		
8. Maintain cricoid pressure until asked to release		

Comments ______________________

____

____

____

Skill Assessment 9-2

Draw Up Medication in a Syringe (Off the Sterile Field)

Student Name ______________________ Date ______________

Instructor ______________________

Procedural Step	Adequate	Needs Review
1. Student is able to provide pertinent information about the medication ordered		
2. Secure the ordered medication and all necessary supplies		
3. Verify that the "five rights" are met		
4. Verify that patient is not allergic to ordered medication		
5. Prepare medication container for withdrawal of medication		
6. Withdraw medication from container		
7. Needle for injection is applied to the syringe		
8. Medication label information is rechecked for accuracy		
9. Medication is labeled according to facility policy		

Comments ______________________

____

____

____

Skill Assessment 9-3

Draw Up Medication in a Syringe (Into the Sterile Field)

Student Name ______________________________ Date ______________

Instructor ____

Procedural Step	Adequate	Needs Review
1. Student is able to provide pertinent information about the medication ordered		
2. Secure the ordered medication and all necessary supplies		
3. Verify that the "five rights" are met		
4. Verify that patient is not allergic to ordered medication		
5. Circulator prepares medication container for withdrawal of medication		
6. STSR and circulator visually and verbally identify medication		
7. STSR withdraws medication from container		
8. STSR and circulator visually and verbally identify medication		
9. Needle for injection is applied to the syringe (if necessary)		
10. Medication is labeled according to facility policy		
11. Medication is passed to surgeon when requested and properly verbally identified		

Comments ____

____

____

____

Skill Assessment 9-4

Accept Medication Into the Sterile Field (Into a Container)

Student Name ______________________ Date ____________

Instructor ______________________

Procedural Step	Adequate	Needs Review
1. Student is able to provide pertinent information about the medication ordered		
2. Secure the ordered medication and all necessary supplies		
3. Verify that the "five rights" are met		
4. Verify that patient is not allergic to ordered medication		
5. Circulator prepares medication for transfer to the sterile field		
6. STSR and circulator visually and verbally identify medication		
7. STSR presents container for acceptance of medication		
8. Medication is transferred to sterile field		
9. STSR and circulator visually and verbally identify medication		
10. Medication is correctly diluted (if necessary)		
11. Medication container is labeled according to facility policy		
12. Medication is prepared for use and additionally labeled (if necessary)		
13. Medication is passed to surgeon when requested and properly verbally identified		

Comments ______________________

____

____

____

CHAPTER 10

Instrumentation, Equipment, and Supplies

OBJECTIVES

After studying this chapter, the reader should be able to:

C 1. Discuss the relationship between instrumentation, equipment, and supplies and quality patient care in the OR.

A 2. Identify items that require sterilization prior to use in the sterile field.

R 3. Identify basic instruments by type, function, and name.

4. Demonstrate proper care, handling, and assembly of instruments.

5. Identify types of special equipment utilized in OR practice and demonstrate proper care, handling techniques, and safety precautions.

6. Identify the names and functions of accessory equipment and demonstrate proper care, handling, and assembly.

7. Identify and prepare supplies used in the OR.

E 8. Discuss the relationship between instruments, equipment, and supplies and the OR environment as related to safety.

Select Key Words

Define the following:

1. ancillary ______
2. aperture ______
3. bipolar electrosurgery ______
4. capillary action ______
5. catheter ______
6. cottonoid ______
7. cryo- ______
8. defibrillator ______
9. drain ______
10. fenestration ______
11. insufflation ______
12. irrigation ______
13. magnification ______
14. monopolar cautery ______
15. Nd:YAG ______
16. pneumatic ______
17. resistance ______
18. retract ______
19. scalpel ______
20. serrations ______
21. stainless steel ______
22. teeth ______
23. tube ______
24. ureteral ______
25. urethral ______

Exercise A – Identification

1. Identify the components of the instrument shown in Figure 10-1.

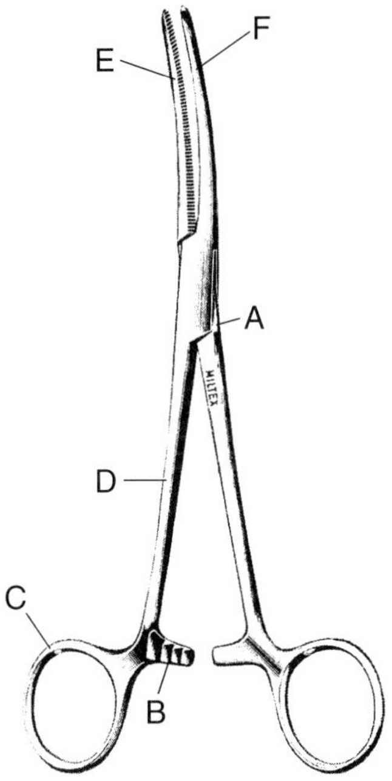

Figure 10-1

A. ____________________

B. ____________________

C.

D. ____________________

E. ____________________

F. ____________________

2. Classify the instruments listed using the following designations:

Accessory Clamping/Occluding Cutting Dilating Grasping/Holding Probing Retracting Suctioning Suturing

A. #3 Knife Handle ____________

B. Allis ____________

C. Babcock ____________

D. Crile ____________

E. Deaver ____________

F. Debakey Tissue Forceps ____________

G. Kocher ____________

H. Metzenbaum ____________

I. Mosquito ____________

J. Needle Holder ____________

K. Poole ____________

L. Richardson ____________

M. Towel Clamp ____________

N. Yankauer ____________

3. Organize the following instruments by size from shortest/smallest to longest/largest.

A. ____________ Crile

B. ____________ Mosquito

C. ____________ Pean

D. ____________ Schnidt

4. A #20 knife blade fits on a # ________ knife handle.

5. A #15 knife blade fits on a # ________ knife handle.

6. An oscillating saw uses a(n) ________ motion.

7. A reciprocating saw uses a(n) ________ motion.

8. The acronym "laser" represents ________

____

9. Trace the path of the electrical current when a unipolar electrosurgical unit is in use by placing the following elements in the correct order.

A. ____________ Active Electrode

B. ____________ Dispersive Electrode

C. ____________ Generator

D. ____________ Generator

E. ____________ Ground

F. ____________ Patient

10. Identify the types of sponges shown in Figure 10-2.

A. ______________________

B. ______________________

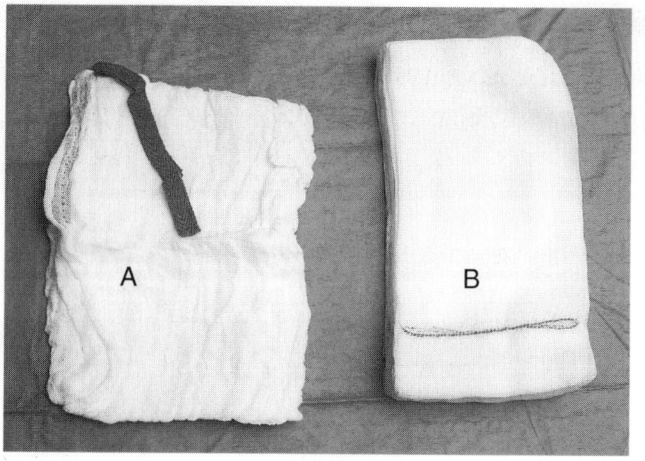

Figure 10-2

Case Studies

☐ CASE STUDY 1

Edward has been assigned to prepare the Cysto Room for a transurethral resection of the prostate (TURP) using the Nd:YAG laser.

1. What does Nd:YAG represent? ______________________

2. What precautions must be taken to protect the patient and staff from the laser beam? ______________________

3. Will the laser be attached to the endoscope?

☐

☐ CASE STUDY 2

Madelena is preparing the OR for a neurosurgical procedure (carpal tunnel release). Both the unipolar and bipolar electrosurgical units are requested on the surgeon's preference card.

1. Will Madelena need two grounding pads (dispersive electrodes)? Why or why not? ______________________

____

____

____

____

2. The patient will be placed in the supine position for the procedure. What anatomic site is the most likely place to affix the grounding pad(s)? ______________________

____

____

____

____

3. The surgeon's preference card requests that a tourniquet be available for the procedure. List at least three items that Madelena will need to facilitate the use of the tourniquet. ______________________

____

____

____

____

☐

Skill Assessment 10-1

Assemble an Instrument Set

Student Name ______________________________ Date ______________

Instructor ____

Procedural Step	Adequate	Needs Review
1. Student is able to state purpose for assembling an instrument set in prescribed manner		
2. Appropriate attire		
3. Wash hands (Standard Precautions)		
4. Equipment and supplies assembled		
5. Organize workspace		
6. Assemble set		
7. Sign/initial count sheet/instrument list		
8. Place internal indicator		
9. Proceed with other tasks		

Comments ____

____

____

____

Skill Assessment 10-2

Instrument Handling – Load, Pass, and Unload a Scalpel Handle

Student Name ______________________ Date ______________

Instructor ______________________

Procedural Step	Adequate	Needs Review
1. Equipment and supplies assembled		
2. Student selects necessary items		
3. Scalpel blade is secured		
4. Blade is applied to handle		
5. Proceed with case preparation or case		
6. Scalpel is held in safe manner		
7. Scalpel is passed or placed for transfer		
8. Scalpel is retrieved		
9. Blade is removed from handle		
10. Discard blade		
11. Proceed with case or case breakdown		

Comments ______________________

Skill Assessment 10-3

Instrument Handling – Recognize, Prepare, and Pass Various Types of Instruments (Sharps, Scissors, Tissue Forceps, Ringed Instruments, and Retractors)

Student Name ______________________________ Date ____________

Instructor ____

Procedural Step	Adequate	Needs Review
1. Equipment and supplies assembled		
2. Mayo stand is set up		
3. Student is able to recognize instruments by name		
4. Student secures instrument requested		
5. Pass sharp instruments or supplies		
6. Pass scissors		
7. Pass tissue forceps		
8. Pass ringed instrument(s)		
9. Pass retractor(s)		
10. Return items to storage location		
11. Attend to other intraoperative actions as needed		

Comments ____

____

____

____

CHAPTER 11

Wound Healing, Sutures, Needles, and Stapling Devices

OBJECTIVES

After studying this chapter, the reader should be able to:

C
1. Define terms relevant to wound healing.
2. List the possible complications of wound healing.

A

3. Explain the classifications of surgical wounds.
4. Define and give examples of types of traumatic wounds.
5. List the factors that influence healing and describe the manner in which they affect the healing process.

R

6. Describe the characteristics of inflammation.
7. List and define common suture terms.
8. Identify suture materials and stapling devices and their usage.
9. Describe the types, characteristics, and uses of natural and synthetic absorbable suture materials.
10. List and describe the common natural and synthetic nonabsorbable sutures, stating their sources, common trade names, and uses.
11. Discuss preparation and handling techniques for suturing and stapling devices, and list the factors relating to the choice of each.
12. List and define common suture techniques.
13. Discuss the basic uses and advantages of stapling instruments.
14. Identify, describe the use of, and demonstrate proper handling of the various types of surgical needles.

E

15. List the types of injury that cause damage to tissues.
16. List the characteristics of the types of healing.
17. Describe the stages/phases of wound healing.

Select Key Terms

Define the following:

1. adhesion ____________________
2. anastomosis ____________________
3. approximated ____________________
4. chromic gut ____________________
5. chronic wound ____________________
6. cicatrix ____________________
7. dead space ____________________
8. debridement ____________________
9. dehiscence ____________________
10. devitalized ____________________
11. evisceration ____________________
12. first intention ____________________
13. fray ____________________
14. French-eyed needle ____________________
15. friable ____________________
16. herniation ____________________
17. immunosuppressed patient ____________________
18. inflammation ____________________
19. laceration ____________________
20. ligate ____________________
21. monofilament ____________________
22. packing ____________________
23. primary suture line ____________________
24. PTFE ____________________
25. second intention ____________________
26. secondary suture line ____________________
27. swaged ____________________
28. tensile strength ____________________
29. third intention ____________________
30. vessel loop ____________________

Case Studies

☐ CASE STUDY 1

James, a 12-year-old male, lost control of his trail bike while riding on a course that he and some friends constructed in a vacant lot. He flew over the handlebars into the dirt onto his left arm. His arm is broken, and the bone is sticking out through the skin. It is 10:00 AM.

1. James has suffered a traumatic injury to his left arm. What classification(s) does his wound fall into?__________

2. James was immediately taken to the Urgent Care Center. It is determined that James will need surgical treatment and will be transferred by ambulance to the nearest hospital, which is 150 miles away. The surgery is scheduled for 4:00 PM. How will the surgical wound be classified? Why?__________

3. Is James at risk for surgical site infection? Why? What steps can be taken to minimize the risk of SSI? __________

☐

☐ CASE STUDY 2

Dorothea just had her ruptured appendix removed. The skin and subcutaneous layers of her wound have been left open. Her surgeon told her that if her wound showed no signs of infection in 5 days he would finish the closure.

1. Why did the surgeon leave the wound partially open? In its present condition, by what method is the wound expected to heal? ______________________

2. What signs will the surgeon use to determine if Dorothea's wound may be closed in 5 days? ______________________

3. If the wound can be closed in 5 days, what type of healing will then be expected? Is the tissue expected to regain normal tensile strength? ______________________

☐

Skill Assessment 11-1

Suture/Needle/Staple Handling – Load, Pass, and Unload a Needle Holder

Student Name ______________________________ Date ______________

Instructor ______________________________

Procedural Step	Adequate	Needs Review
1. Equipment and supplies assembled		
2. Select necessary items		
3. Open suture packet		
4. Needle holder is applied		
5. Suture is removed from packet		
6. Pass suture		
7. Companion instruments passed		
8. Suture is retrieved		
9. Needle holder is unloaded		
10. Return items to storage location		
11. Attend to other intraoperative actions as needed		

Comments ______________________________

____

____

____

Skill Assessment 11-2

Suture/Needle/Staple Handling – Load Empty Needle, Thread Suture, Pass, and Reload

Student Name ______________________________ Date ______________

Instructor ______________________________

Procedural Step	Adequate	Needs Review
1. Equipment and supplies assembled		
2. Select necessary items		
3. Open suture packet		
4. Needle is placed in needle holder		
5. Needle holder is moved to left hand		
6. Suture is threaded		
7. Pass suture		
8. Companion instruments passed		
9. Needle is retrieved		
10. Reset needle and reload (if necessary)		
11. Needle holder is unloaded		
12. Return items to storage location		
13. Attend to other intraoperative actions as needed		

Comments ______________________________

____

____

____

Skill Assessment 11-3

Suture/Needle/Staple Handling – Pass Ties (Includes Reel, Free Ties, and Ties on a Pass)

Student Name ______________________________ Date ______________

Instructor ____

Procedural Step	Adequate	Needs Review
1. Equipment and supplies assembled		
2. Select necessary items		
3. Prepare, pass, and retrieve reel		
4. Prepare and pass free tie		
5. Prepare and pass tie on a pass		
6. Attend to other intraoperative actions as needed		

Comments ____

____

____

____

Skill Assessment 11-4

Suture/Needle/Staple Handling – Load, Pass, and Unload Various Types of Stapling/Clipping Devices

Student Name ______________________ Date ____________

Instructor ______________________

Procedural Step	Adequate	Needs Review
1. Equipment and supplies assembled		
2. Select necessary items		
3. Item is prepared for use		
4. Item is passed		
5. Item is retrieved		
6. Attend to other intraoperative actions as needed		

Comments ______________________

CHAPTER 12

Surgical Case Management

OBJECTIVES

After studying this chapter, the reader should be able to:

C 1. Describe the role of the STSR in caring for the surgical patient.

A 2. Demonstrate techniques of opening and preparing supplies and instruments needed for any operative procedure with the maintenance of sterile technique at all times.

3. Demonstrate the proper techniques for the surgical hand scrub, gowning, gloving, and assisting team members.

4. Demonstrate the proper technique for preparing supplies and instruments on a sterile field.

R 5. Demonstrate and explain in detail the procedure for counting instruments, sponges, needles, and other items on the sterile field.

6. Demonstrate the initial steps for starting a procedure.

7. Demonstrate intraoperative handling of sterile equipment and supplies.

E 8. Explain and demonstrate postoperative routines.

Select Key Terms

Define the following:

1. adhesive ______________________
2. anticipate ______________________
3. antimicrobial ______________________
4. biohazard ______________________
5. circumferentially ______________________
6. count ______________________
7. craniotomy ______________________
8. cylindrical ______________________
9. donning ______________________
10. foreign body ______________________
11. handwash ______________________
12. indicator ______________________
13. lap sponge ______________________
14. mask ______________________
15. neutral zone ______________________
16. pathology ______________________
17. PPE ______________________
18. resident organisms ______________________
19. scrub (sterile) attire ______________________
20. sterile team member ______________________
21. stockinette ______________________
22. surgeon's preference card ______________________
23. surgical scrub ______________________
24. transient organisms ______________________
25. wraparound-style gown ______________________

Case Studies

CASE STUDY 1

Sean is a student STSR for an LAVH. As he reaches for a supply item being handed by the circulator, his left glove touches the outside of the packet.

1. Does Sean have a problem? What is it?

2. What steps need to be taken to correct the problem?

3. Describe the procedure(s) for changing a contaminated glove.

☐ CASE STUDY 2

It is LuAnn's big day. She is scrubbing her first case as a student. She wants desperately to do everything right.

1. What type of surgical scrub should LuAnn perform? Why?

2. Describe the counted brush stroke method for a surgical scrub.

3. Which method of self-gloving will LuAnn use after she has donned her sterile gown? Why?

☐

Skill Assessment 12-1

OR Attire

Student Name ______________________________ Date ______________

Instructor ____

Procedural Step	Adequate	Needs Review
1. Student is able to state purpose for wearing OR attire		
2. Student is able to state situations when variations in OR attire may occur		
3. Student is able to state when OR attire is to be worn		
4. Scrub suit		
5. No jewelry		
6. No cosmetics		
7. Hair cover		
8. Identification		
9. Radiation monitoring device		
10. Shoes appropriate to OR		
11. Shoe covers		
12. Mask		
13. Eyewear		

Comments ____

____

____

____

Skill Assessment 12-2

Open Sterile Supplies – Back Table Pack

Student Name ______________________________ Date ______________

Instructor ______________________________

Procedural Step	Adequate	Needs Review
1. Appropriate attire		
2. Wash hands (Standard Precautions)		
3. Equipment and supplies assembled		
4. Check integrity of package		
5. Remove dust cover		
6. Check integrity of inner package		
7. Orient pack on back table		
8. Open first fold and remove accessory items, if present		
9. Open second fold		
10. Open third fold		
11. Reposition self to open fourth fold		
12. Open fourth fold		
13. Proceed with case preparation		

Comments ______________________________

Skill Assessment 12-3

Open Sterile Supplies – Small Wrapped Package (Such as Initial Gown – On Clean Surface)

Student Name ______________________ Date ______________

Instructor ______________________

Procedural Step	Adequate	Needs Review
1. Appropriate attire		
2. Wash hands (Standard Precautions)		
3. Equipment and supplies assembled		
4. Check integrity of package		
5. Orient package on appropriate surface		
6. Open first fold		
7. Open second fold		
8. Open third fold		
9. Open fourth fold		
10. Proceed with case preparation		

Comments ______________________

Skill Assessment 12-4

Open Sterile Supplies – Small Wrapped Package (Onto Sterile Field or Secured by STSR)

Student Name ______________________________ Date ______________

Instructor ______________________________

Procedural Step	Adequate	Needs Review
1. Appropriate attire		
2. Wash hands (Standard Precautions)		
3. Equipment and supplies assembled		
4. Check integrity of package		
5. Orient package properly in hand		
6. Open first fold, secure flap		
7. Open second fold, secure flap		
8. Open third fold, secure flap		
9. Open fourth fold, secure flap		
10. Approach sterile field/STSR		
11. Transfer item to sterile field/STSR		
12. Discard wrapper		
13. Proceed with case preparation		

Comments ______________________________

Skill Assessment 12-5

Open Sterile Supplies – Peel Pack

Student Name ______________________________ Date ______________

Instructor ____

Procedural Step	Adequate	Needs Review
1. Appropriate attire		
2. Wash hands (Standard Precautions)		
3. Equipment and supplies assembled		
4. Check integrity of package		
5. Orient package properly in both hands		
6. Slowly pull sides of peel pack away from each other		
7. Continue opening package		
8. Approach sterile field/STSR		
9. Transfer item to sterile field/STSR		
10. Discard wrapper		
11. Proceed with case preparation		

Comments ____

____

____

____

Skill Assessment 12-6

Open Sterile Supplies – Instrument Set (Container System)

Student Name ______________________________ Date ______________

Instructor ____

Procedural Step	Adequate	Needs Review
1. Appropriate attire		
2. Wash hands (Standard Precautions)		
3. Equipment and supplies assembled		
4. Check integrity of container		
5. Place instrument container on suitable surface		
6. Remove seals		
7. Release lid		
8. Lift lid		
9. Inspect interior of container		
10. Inspect lid		
11. Set lid in convenient location		
12. Proceed with case preparation		

Comments ____

Skill Assessment 12-7

Open Sterile Supplies – Pour Sterile Solution

Student Name ______________________________ Date ______________

Instructor ______________________________

Procedural Step	Adequate	Needs Review
1. Student is able to provide pertinent information about the sterile solution ordered		
2. Appropriate attire		
3. Wash hands (Standard Precautions)		
4. Equipment and supplies assembled		
5. Verify that the "five rights" are met		
6. Verify patient allergy status		
7. Remove protective outer seal from solution container		
8. Remove inner seal		
9. Approach sterile field		
10. STSR and circulator visually and verbally identify solution		
11. Pour sterile solution		
12. STSR and circulator visually and verbally identify solution		
13. Proceed with case preparation		

Comments ______________________________

Skill Assessment 12-8

Surgical Scrub – Counted Brush Stroke Method

Student Name ______________________________ Date ______________

Instructor ______________________________

Procedural Step	Adequate	Needs Review
1. Student is able to define surgical scrub		
2. Student is able to state purpose for performing surgical scrub		
3. Appropriate attire		
4. Equipment and supplies are assembled		
5. Inspect integrity of hands and arms		
6. Open brush package		
7. Turn on water and adjust temperature		
8. Wet hands and arms, apply soap, lather		
9. Clean nails		
10. Rinse		
11. Secure and prepare brush		
12. Scrub nails of first hand		
13. Scrub fingers of first hand		
14. Scrub hand of first arm		
15. Scrub arm to 2″ above elbow of first arm		
16. Transfer brush to scrubbed hand and scrub opposite extremity		
17. Discard brush		
18. Rinse		
19. Proceed to OR		

Comments ______________________________

Skill Assessment 12-9

Gown – Self
(Dry, Don Gown and Gloves – Closed Glove Technique)

Student Name ______________________ Date ______________

Instructor ______________________

Procedural Step	Adequate	Needs Review
1. Enter OR		
2. Secure towel		
3. Open towel		
4. Dry first hand and arm		
5. Transfer towel to opposite hand		
6. Dry opposite hand		
7. Discard towel		
8. Secure gown		
9. Unfold gown		
10. Don gown		
11. Secure first glove		
12. Position glove appropriately		
13. Don first glove		
14. Secure and don second glove		
15. Wrap around back of gown		
16. Remove lubricant (powder) from gloves		
17. Proceed with case preparation		

Comments ______________________

Skill Assessment 12-10

Gown – Assist a Team Member (Pass Towel, Apply Gown and Gloves – Open Glove Technique)

Student Name ______________________________ Date ______________

Instructor ____

Procedural Step	Adequate	Needs Review
1. Prepare items in advance of need		
2. Secure towel		
3. Open towel		
4. Present towel to team member		
5. Secure gown		
6. Unfold gown		
7. Present gown		
8. Secure right glove		
9. Prepare right glove		
10. Present right glove		
11. Secure, prepare, and present left glove		
12. Wrap around back of gown		
13. Remove lubricant (powder) from gloves		
14. Proceed with case preparation or case		

Comments ____

Skill Assessment 12-11

Disrobe
(To Replace Sterile Attire During Case)

Student Name ______________________ Date ____________

Instructor ______________________

Procedural Step	Adequate	Needs Review
1. Recognize that gloves and/or gown are contaminated during case		
2. Step away from sterile field and request new gown and appropriate size gloves		
3. Remain still, with back to circulator while gown is unfastened		
4. Face circulator; remain still while gown is removed		
5. Turn hands palm up and present one at a time to circulator (usually right hand first)		
6. Apply sterile gown and gloves		
7. Return to sterile field and continue with tasks		

Comments ______________________

____

____

____

Skill Assessment 12-12

Disrobe
(End of Case)

Student Name ______________________ Date ____________

Instructor ______________________

Procedural Step	Adequate	Needs Review
1. All tasks that require gown and gloves are complete		
2. Back of gown is unfastened		
3. Grasp gown near shoulders and roll away from self		
4. Remove gown (place gown in proper receptacle if feasible)		
5. Remove soiled gloves		
6. Grasp palm of glove to be removed first with opposite hand		
7. Remove first glove		
8. Keep removed glove in hand that remains gloved		
9. Begin to remove second glove		
10. Contain first glove inside of inverted second glove		
11. Finish removal of second glove		
12. Properly dispose of gown and gloves		
13. Wash hands (Standard Precautions)		

Comments ______________________

Skill Assessment 12-13

Dress the Mayo Stand

Student Name ______________________ Date ______________

Instructor ______________________

Procedural Step	Adequate	Needs Review
1. Equipment and supplies assembled		
2. Orient Mayo stand cover		
3. Insert hands in cuff of Mayo stand cover		
4. Secure folded edges of Mayo stand cover		
5. Approach Mayo stand		
6. Insert bare Mayo stand into prepared pocket of Mayo stand cover		
7. Slide Mayo stand cover onto Mayo stand		
8. Allow Mayo stand cover to unfold over back edge of stand		
9. Make final adjustments		
10. Place towels		
11. Proceed with case preparation		

Comments ______________________

Skill Assessment 12-14

Fill a Bulb Syringe

Student Name ______________________________ Date ______________

Instructor ______________________________

Procedural Step	Adequate	Needs Review
1. Equipment and supplies assembled		
2. Prepare bulb syringe		
3. Remove air		
4. Fill bulb syringe		
5. Proceed with case preparation or case		

Comments ______________________________

____

____

____

Skill Assessment 12-15

Remove Instrument Set from Container

Student Name ______________________________ Date ______________

Instructor ____

Procedural Step	Adequate	Needs Review
1. Equipment and supplies assembled		
2. Approach instrument container		
3. Secure instrument basket		
4. Step away from instrument container		
5. Place instrument basket on back table		
6. Proceed with case preparation or case		

Comments ____

____

____

____

Skill Assessment 12-16

Case Management – Pre-Case Preparation (Prior to Scrub)

Student Name ______________________________ Date ______________

Instructor ____

Procedural Step	Adequate	Needs Review
1. Appropriate attire		
2. Wash hands (Standard Precautions)		
3. Assignment received		
4. Secure surgeon preference card		
5. Locate case cart or assemble necessary items		
6. Verify that all items are present		
7. OR prepared for use		
8. Sterile items placed for use		
9. Open standard and specialty items		
10. Double-check supplies		
11. Proceed with case preparation		

Comments ____

Skill Assessment 12-17

Case Management – Case Preparation (Beginning with Surgical Scrub)

Student Name ______________________________ Date ______________

Instructor ______________________________

Procedural Step	Adequate	Needs Review
1. Appropriate attire		
2. Sterility is maintained at all times		
3. Perform surgical scrub		
4. Proceed to OR		
5. Approach sterile field, secure towel, and dry self		
6. Don sterile gown		
7. Apply sterile gloves		
8. Prepare back table and basin set; dress Mayo stand		
9. Count necessary items		
10. Mayo stand prepared for use		
11. Preparation time less than 20 minutes		

Comments ______________________________

____

____

____

Skill Assessment 12-18

Case Management – Drape (Basic Laparotomy)

Student Name ____________________ Date ____________

Instructor ____________________

Procedural Step	Adequate	Needs Review
1. Equipment and supplies assembled		
2. Prepare drape materials		
3. Remain vigilant		
4. Report and correct problems immediately		
5. Hold drape materials at correct level		
6. Pass drape materials correctly		
7. Move safely between sterile fields		
8. Hand drapes in proper sequence		
9. Protect hands with drape cuff		
10. Communicate with team members as needed		
11. Other equipment is ready for placement		
12. Move furniture into position		
13. Proceed with case preparation or case		

Comments ____________________

Skill Assessment 12-19

Case Management – Intraoperative Actions

Student Name ______________________________ Date ______________

Instructor ______________________________

Procedural Step	Adequate	Needs Review
1. Equipment and supplies assembled		
2. Assist other team members to enter sterile field		
3. Perform tasks related to draping		
4. Place additional equipment on field as needed		
5. Move furniture into position		
6. Prepare field		
7. Pass scalpel		
8. Handle electrosurgical pencil properly		
9. Hand instruments correctly		
10. Prepare, identify, and handle all solutions correctly		
11. Prepare, identify, and handle all medications correctly		
12. Remove small sponges (if necessary)		
13. Respond to team member needs appropriately		
14. Communicate effectively with circulator		
15. Prepare, identify, and handle sutures and needles correctly		
16. Perform closing count(s)		
17. Report and correct problems immediately		
18. Maintain an orderly field		
19. Prepare for end of case		
20. Maintain sterile field until patient removed from OR		
21. Proceed with post-procedure actions		

Comments ______________________________

Skill Assessment 12-20

Case Management – Post-Procedure Actions

Student Name ______________________________ Date ______________

Instructor ____

Procedural Step	Adequate	Needs Review
1. Maintain sterile field until patient removed from OR		
2. Remove drapes from patient		
3. Assist with patient care as needed		
4. Return to tasks related to breakdown of field		
5. Handle all materials safely		
6. Dispose of all sharps correctly		
7. Handle all biohazardous waste (linen and trash) correctly		
8. Follow policy for instrument care		
9. Remove gown and gloves properly		
10. Wash hands (Standard Precautions)		
11. Care for equipment as needed		
12. Follow OR cleaning/turn-over procedure		

Comments ____

____

____

____

CHAPTER 13

Diagnostic Procedures

OBJECTIVES

After studying this chapter, the reader should be able to:

A 1. Apply knowledge of anatomy and physiology to determine which diagnostic examinations will be useful.

P 2. List the sources of patient data.

3. List and discuss techniques used to establish the diagnosis.

O 4. Determine which diagnostic procedures will require surgical intervention.

5. Identify the major indications for surgical intervention.

S 6. Understand the surgical technologist's role in caring for each specific type of specimen.

Select Key Terms

Define the following:

1. angina ______
2. auscultation ______
3. biopsy ______
4. capnography ______
5. C-arm ______
6. cholangiography ______
7. contrast media ______
8. CSF ______
9. cystoscopy ______
10. ECG ______
11. EEG ______
12. frozen section ______
13. -gram ______
14. Gram stain ______
15. -graph ______
16. indwelling ______
17. isotope scanning ______
18. obstruction ______
19. palpation ______
20. prosthesis ______
21. Roentgenography ______
22. sign ______
23. symptom ______
24. urinalysis (UA) ______
25. ultrasonography ______

Exercise A – Anatomy

1. Identify the structures of the biliary tract shown in Figure 13-1.

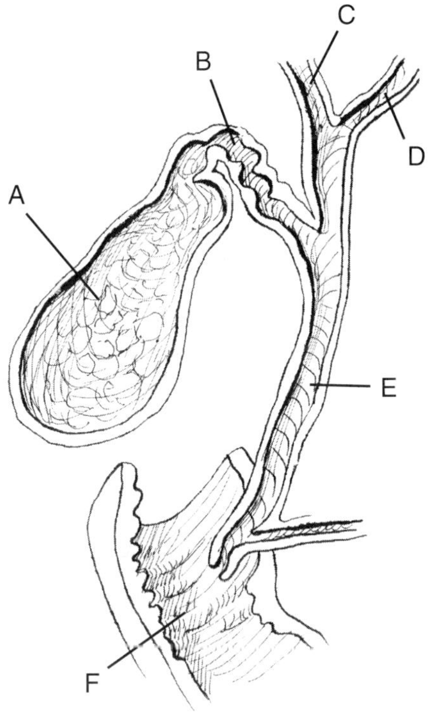

Figure 13-1

A. ______________ B. ______________

C. ______________ D. ______________

E. ______________ F. ______________

2. What type of radiographic exam would be used to visualize the structures of the biliary tract?

____

____

3. Identify the bony structures shown in Figure 13-2.

A. ______________ B. ______________

C. ______________ D. ______________

E. ______________ F. ______________

4. What radiographic view is shown in Figure 13-2, and which structure(s) is/are the primary focus of the exam? ______________________________

____

____

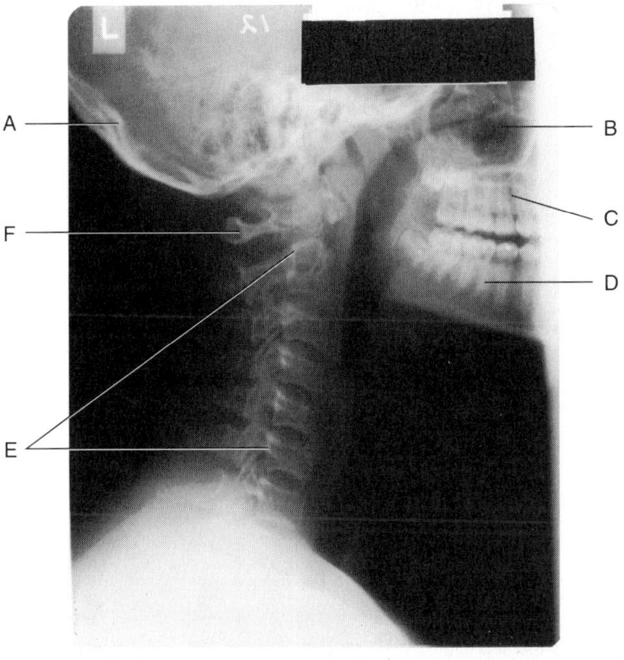

Figure 13-2

5. Identify the bony structures shown in Figure 13-3.

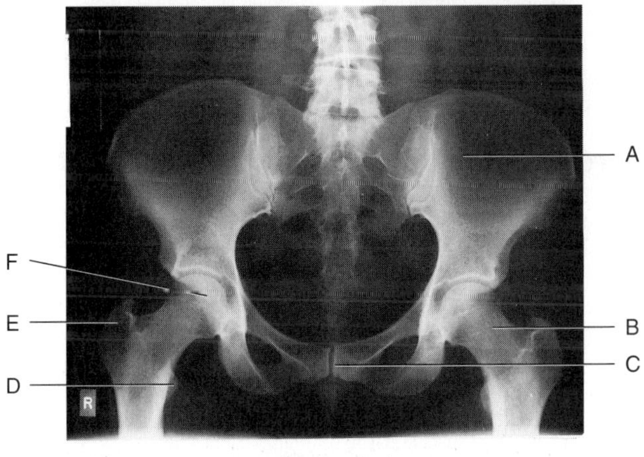

Figure 13-3

A. ______________ B. ______________

C. ______________ D. ______________

E. ______________ F. ______________

6. What radiographic view is shown in Figure 13-3?

____

____

7. In what position was the patient placed in order to obtain the radiographic view shown in Figure 13-3?

____

____

8. Identify the structures of the urinary system shown in Figure 13-4.

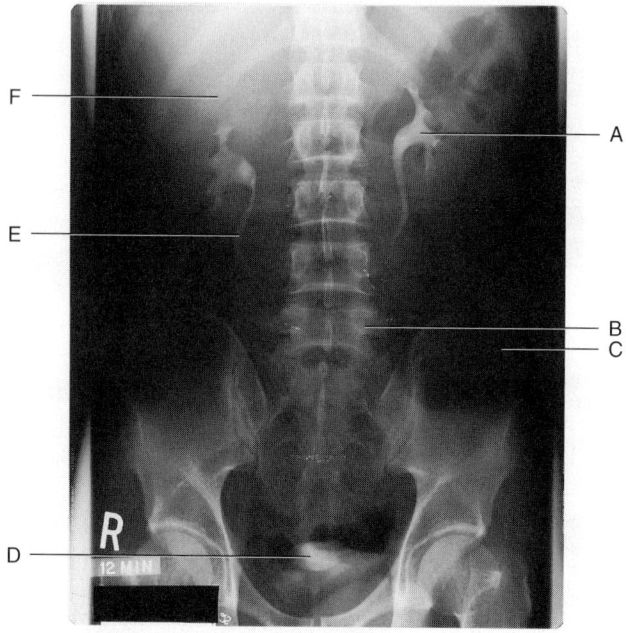

Figure 13-4

A. ________________ B. ________________

C. ________________ D. ________________

E. ________________ F. ________________

9. Has contrast been used to obtain the radiograph shown in Figure 13-4? ______________________

____

____

10. In what position was the patient placed in order to obtain the radiographic view shown in Figure 13-4?

____

____

11. Figure 13-5 shows an image of the liver. How was this image obtained? ______________________

____

____

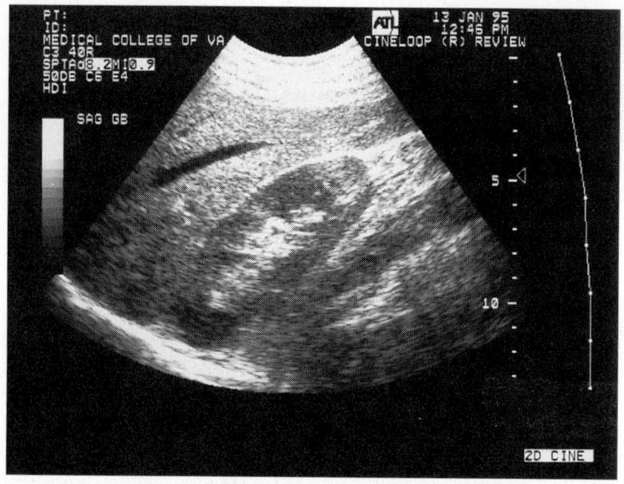

Figure 13-5

12. Why is ultrasonography ideal for examination of the fetus? ______________________

____

____

13. What piece of radiographic equipment is shown in Figure 13-6? ______________________

____

____

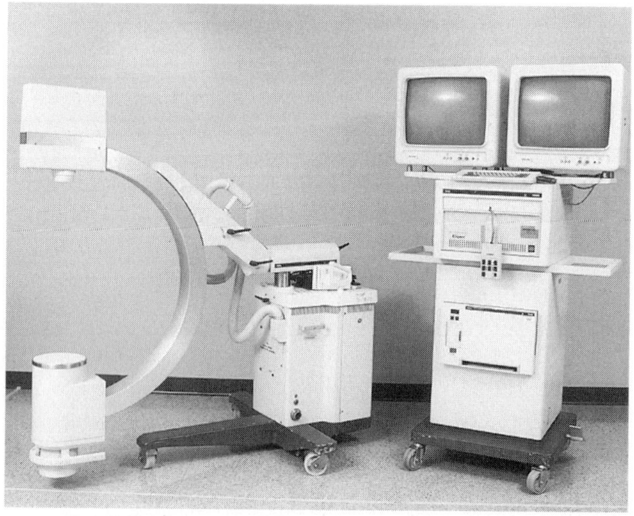

Figure 13-6

14. What is the advantage of fluoroscopy? ______________________

____

____

15. Locate the following structures in the correct abdominal quadrant.

RUQ = Right Upper Quadrant	LUQ = Left Upper Quadrant
RLQ = Right Lower Quadrant	LLQ = Left Lower Quadrant
A. Gallbladder_______	B. Spleen_______
C. Appendix_______	D. Liver_______
E. Stomach_______	F. Left Ovary_______

Exercise B – Pathology

1. What pathologic condition(s) is/are detected with the use of cholecystography? ______________________

2. What type of examination is necessary to identify a pneumothorax? ______________________

3. What type of examination(s) would a patient experiencing a possible ureteral obstruction undergo to confirm the diagnosis? ______________________

4. What is the one condition that an MIBG scan is useful in diagnosing? ______________________

5. Will pressure readings from a Swan-Ganz catheter placed in the pulmonary artery be useful in diagnosing pulmonary embolism? ______________________

6. What is the purpose of performing a Gram stain? __

7. The patient is suspected to have a spinal cord tumor. Will an MRI or a CT scan be more useful in visualizing the soft tissue tumor? ______________________

8. What is considered the first step in determining the etiology of a patient's condition? Why? ______________________

9. Three types of visualization may be used by the examiner during a physical exam. Name the three types, explain how they differ, list any special equipment that may be needed for each, and give at least one example of each type.

   A. ______________________

   B. ______________________

   C. ______________________

10. To confirm a preliminary diagnosis of deep vein thrombosis, what diagnostic examination will be ordered by the physician? ______________________

11. A bone scan is an example of what type of scan? The term *hot spot* refers to what aspect of the scan, and what condition might be indicated by its presence? ______________________

12. Name the two methods of administering radiation therapy. What is the purpose of administering radiation therapy? ______________________

13. The physician has ordered a blood gas study. Will the blood be drawn from a venous or arterial source? ______

14. What is the normal amount of glucose expected in a urine sample? Use Table 13-3 from the textbook to determine your answer. ______

15. A "culture and sensitivity" has been ordered. The organism has been "cultured" and identified. What is determined by the "sensitivity" portion of the exam?

Exercise C – Operation

1. Name the five types of cholecystography.

   A. ______ B. ______

   C. ______ D. ______

   E. ______

2. What purpose does a "scout" film (X-ray) serve?

3. Is transesophageal echocardiography an invasive procedure? Why? ______

4. What does the term *noninvasive* mean?

5. What is the ideal location for insertion of a Swan-Ganz pulmonary artery catheter? List two alternative locations. ______

6. List four intraoperative applications for fluoroscopy.

   A. ______

   B. ______

   C. ______

   D. ______

7. Explain the difference(s) between incisional biopsy and excisional biopsy. ______

8. The surgeon has requested that fluid aspirated from the thoracic cavity be sent to the laboratory to be cultured for aerobic and anaerobic organisms. What special supplies (if any) will be needed? ______

9. The surgeon has requested a frozen section on a piece of breast tissue that has been excised. Will the specimen be placed in formalin? Why?

10. Why is it necessary for the pathologist to be readily available to perform a frozen section?

11. A six-month-old is scheduled to undergo a CT scan with general anesthesia. What is the most likely reason that general anesthesia will be administered? ______

12. Explain the difference between a diagnostic and a therapeutic procedure. ______

13. List the steps, in order, for percutaneous placement of a femoral artery catheter using the Seldinger technique.

A. ______

B. ______

C. ______

D. ______

E. ______

F. ______

G. ______

H. ______

14. What is the difference between a simple voided urine specimen and a clean-catch specimen? What supplies are needed for each? ______

15. Panendoscopy of the upper aerodigestive tract has been scheduled. What structures will be visualized, and what, if any, specialized equipment will be needed? ______

Exercise D – Specific Variations

Student Name ______________________ Date ____________

Instructor ______________________

Surgical Procedure – Student Case Study Report

The student will be provided with basic patient information (real or simulated) and is expected to complete the following case study.

1. Procedure name: ____________
2. Definition of procedure: ____________
3. What is the purpose of the procedure? ____________
4. What is the expected outcome of the procedure?
5. Patient age: ____________
6. Gender: ____________
7. Additional pertinent patient information: ____________
8. Probable preoperative diagnosis: ____________
9. How was the diagnosis determined? ____________
10. Discuss the relevant anatomy. ____________
11. List the general and procedure-specific equipment that will be needed for the procedure.

12. List the general and procedure-specific instruments that will be needed for the procedure.

13. List the basic and procedure-specific supplies that will be needed for the procedure.

Pack

Basin

Gloves

Blades

Drapes

Drains

Dressings

Suture–Type of Suture, Needle (if applicable), and Anticipated Tissue Usage

Pharmaceuticals

Miscellaneous

14. Operative preparation:

15. What type of anesthesia will likely be used? Why?

16. List any special anesthesia equipment that may be needed.

17. Patient position during the procedure:

18. What supplies will be necessary for positioning?

19. What type of shave/skin preparation will be necessary (if any)?

20. Define the anatomic perimeters of the prep.

21. List the order in which the drapes will be applied, and describe any specific variations.

22. List any practical considerations.

23. List the procedural steps, and describe the preparatory and supportive actions of the STSR during each step (use additional space if necessary).

Operative Procedure	Technical Considerations
1.	•
	•
2.	•
	•
3.	•
	•
4.	•
	•
5.	•
	•

Operative Procedure *(continued)*	Technical Considerations *(continued)*
6.	•
	•
7.	•
	•
8.	•
	•
9.	•
	•
10.	•
	•

24. What is the postoperative diagnosis?______________

25. Describe the immediate postoperative care.

26. What is the patient's long-term prognosis?

27. What are the possible complications?______________

28. Comments or questions:______________

29. What is the most valuable information you obtained from preparing this surgical procedure case study?

Case Studies

☐ CASE STUDY 1

Paul, a young athlete, has been scheduled for surgical removal of a Baker's cyst.

1. What is a Baker's cyst?

2. What diagnostic radiographic exam may have been performed to diagnose Paul's cyst?

3. In what position will Paul be placed to remove the Baker's cyst?

☐

☐ CASE STUDY 2

Lynn has just suffered a fall off a stepladder. She fell backwards, striking her head against the wall. She temporarily lost consciousness but is now awake, alert, and oriented. Lynn was transferred to the emergency department at the local hospital by ambulance with a cervical collar in place. She responds appropriately to verbal commands and is able to move all four extremities.

1. Lynn is complaining that the collar is too tight. Should it be removed? Why?

____

____

____

____

2. What diagnostic examination must be performed prior to removal of the cervical collar?

____

____

____

____

3. What type of physician specialist will be needed to interpret the results of the diagnostic exam?

____

____

____

____

____

☐

CHAPTER 14 General Surgery

OBJECTIVES

After studying this chapter, the reader should be able to:

A 1. Discuss the relevant anatomy and physiology of the abdominal wall, digestive system, hepatic and biliary system, pancreas, spleen, thyroid, and breast.

P 2. Describe the pathology and related terminology of each system or organ that prompts surgical intervention.

3. Discuss any preoperative diagnostic procedures and tests.

4. Discuss any special preoperative preparation procedures related to general surgery procedures.

O 5. Identify the names and uses of general surgery instruments, supplies, and drugs.

6. Identify the names and uses of special equipment related to general surgery.

7. Discuss the intraoperative preparation of the patient undergoing a general surgical procedure.

8. Define and give an overview of illustrative general surgery procedures.

9. Discuss the purpose and expected outcomes of the illustrative procedures.

10. Discuss the immediate postoperative care and possible complications of the illustrative procedures.

S 11. Discuss any specific variations related to the preoperative, intraoperative, and postoperative care of the general surgery patient.

Select Key Terms

Define the following:

1. absorption ______

2. anastomosis ______

3. ascites ______

4. bile ______

5. chole- ______

6. chyle ______

7. chyme ______

8. -cysto ______

9. -docho- ______

10. -ectomy ______

11. excision ______

12. incision ______

13. lysis ______

14. necrosis ______

15. -oma ______

16. -ostomy ______

17. -otomy ______

18. parietal ______

19. peristalsis ______

20. peritoneum ______

21. portal venous system ______

22. -stasis ______

23. stenosis ______

24. ulcer ______

25. viscera ______

Exercise A – Anatomy

1. Trace the alimentary pathway by placing the following elements in the correct order.

A. ______________________ Anus

B. ______________________ Ascending colon

C. ______________________ Body of stomach

D. ______________________ Cardia of stomach

E. ______________________ Cardiac sphincter

F. ______________________ Cecum

G. ______________________ Descending colon

H. ______________________ Duodenum

I. ______________________ Epiglottis

J. ______________________ Esophagus

K. ______________________ Fundus of stomach

L. ______________________ Hepatic flexure

M. ______________________ Ileocecal valve

N. ______________________ Ileum

O. ______________________ Jejunum

P. ______________________ Labia

Q. ______________________ Mouth

R. ______________________ Pharynx

S. ______________________ Pyloric sphincter

T. ______________________ Pylorus of stomach

U. ______________________ Rectum

V. ______________________ Sigmoid colon

W. ______________________ Splenic flexure

X. ______________________ Transverse colon

Y. ______________________ Uvula

2. Identify the accessory digestive ducts and organs shown in Figure 14-1.

A. ________________ B. ________________

C. ________________ D. ________________

E. ________________ F. ________________

G. ________________ H. ________________

I. ________________ J. ________________

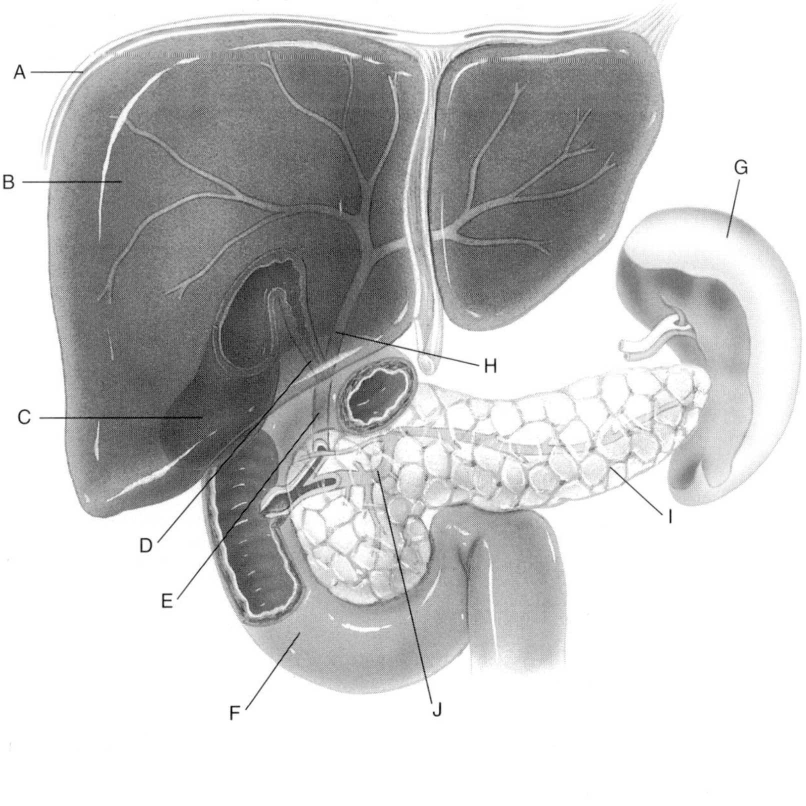

Figure 14-1

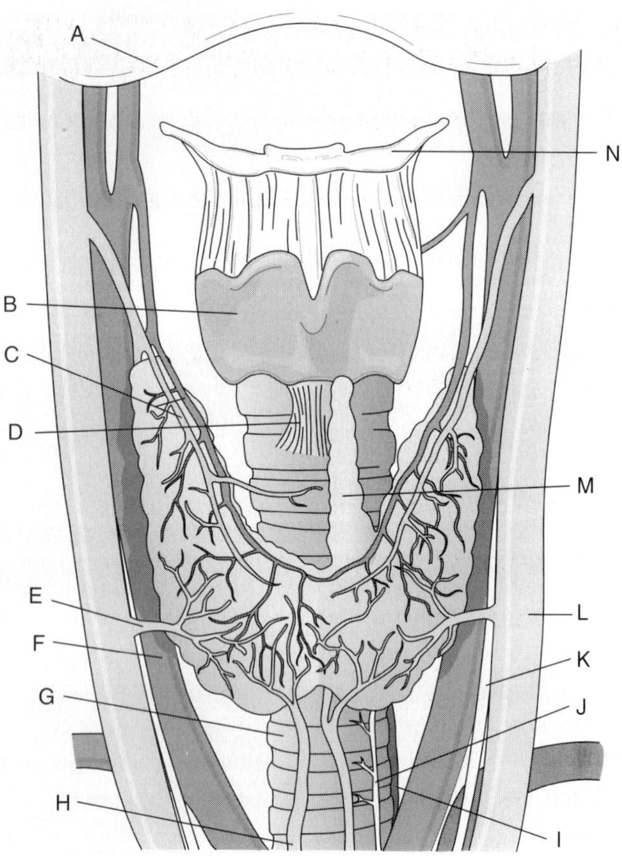

Figure 14-2

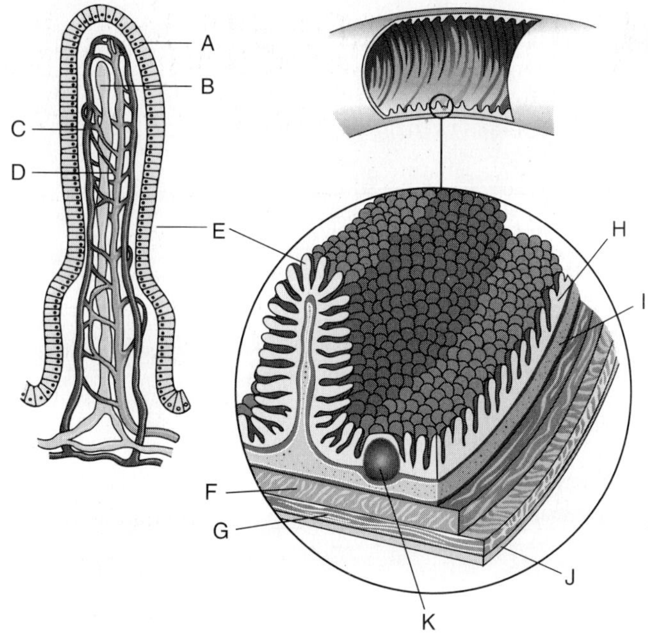

Figure 14-3

3. Identify the structures of the thyroid gland shown in Figure 14-2.

A. ________ B. ________
C. ________ D. ________
E. ________ F. ________
G. ________ H. ________
I. ________ J. ________
K. ________ L. ________
M. ________ N. ________

4. Identify the components of the intestinal wall shown in Figure 14-3.

A. ________ B. ________
C. ________ D. ________
E. ________ F. ________
G. ________ H. ________
I. ________ J. ________
K. ________

5. The gallbladder is located in the ________ ________ quadrant of the abdomen.

6. Linea alba literally means ________ ________ and will be found in the ________ abdominal wall.

7. Parasympathetic innervation to the stomach is provided by the ________ nerve.

8. The four layers of the wall of the colon are ________, ________, ________, and ________.

9. The pancreas is classified as both a(n) ________ and ________ gland.

10. What is the primary function of the peritoneum?

____

____

11. Name the five sections of the stomach.

A. ________
B. ________
C. ________
D. ________
E. ________

12. Where are the islets of Langerhans located, and what is their function? ________________

13. What is the largest organ in the normal abdominal cavity? ________________

14. List the functions that are performed by the cells of the liver.

A. ________________

B. ________________

C. ________________

D. ________________

E. ________________

F. ________________

15. What is the function of the sphincter of Oddi?

Exercise B – Pathology

1. Peptic ulcers are most frequently found in which location? ________________

2. Explain the difference between an incarcerated and a strangulated hernia. ________________

3. Is a direct hernia congenital or acquired? ________________

4. What is diverticulitis? ________________

5. What causes intra-abdominal adhesions? ________________

6. Are a hemorrhoid and a pile the same? ________________

7. What are the two types of choleliths, and what is the composition of each?

A. ________________

B. ________________

8. What is "referred" pain? ________________

9. What is the usual cause of appendicitis? ________________

10. Thrombocytopenia is a deficiency of __________ in the blood.

11. Which diagnostic tools will be useful in determining liver pathology? ________________

12. List four of the causes of varicose veins of the lower extremity.

A. ________________

B. ________________

C. ________________

D. ________________

13. Define gynecomastia, and describe the surgical treatment that may be recommended to treat the condition. ________________

14. Overactivity of the thyroid gland is referred to as ________________

15. What is meant by the term *staging* in reference to malignant tumors? ______

Exercise C – Operation

1. Laparoscopic Nissen fundoplication is performed to treat which condition(s)? ______

2. What structure is dilated with a Maloney dilator? Is the Maloney dilator inserted under sterile conditions? Why? ______

3. List two reasons for performing a gastrostomy.

   A. ______

   B. ______

4. Explain what is meant by the phrase "mobilize the bowel."

5. List the three basic configurations for intestinal anastomosis.

   A. ______

   B. ______

   C. ______

6. Describe the technique used to care for instrumentation and supplies that have been exposed to the inside of the intestinal tract.

7. What is a stoma? ______

8. What is the purpose of a T-tube, and where is it placed? ______

9. Why is it important to expel all air from the cholangiogram system prior to an intraoperative cholangiogram? ______

10. What is the reason for providing a second setup to perform a breast reconstruction following a modified radical mastectomy due to a malignancy? ______

11. Why is it important for the STSR to maintain the sterile field until the patient is extubated and breathing freely following a thyroidectomy?

12. What instruments and supplies will be needed to enter the common bile duct for CBDE? ______

13. Name the two positions that provide access to the anus.

    A. ______

    B. ______

14. What type of procedure is performed through a McBurney's incision? ______

15. McVay repair is performed to correct which condition? ______

Exercise D – Specific Variations

Student Name ______________________ Date ______________

Instructor ______________________________

Surgical Procedure – Student Case Study Report

The student will be provided with basic patient information (real or simulated) and is expected to complete the following case study.

1. Procedure name: ______________________
2. Definition of procedure: ______________________
3. What is the purpose of the procedure? ______________________
4. What is the expected outcome of the procedure?
5. Patient age: ______________________
6. Gender: ______________________
7. Additional pertinent patient information: ______________________
8. Probable preoperative diagnosis: ______________________
9. How was the diagnosis determined? ______________________
10. Discuss the relevant anatomy. ______________________
11. List the general and procedure-specific equipment that will be needed for the procedure.

12. List the general and procedure-specific instruments that will be needed for the procedure.

13. List the basic and procedure-specific supplies that will be needed for the procedure.

Pack

Basin

Gloves

Blades

Drapes

Drains

Dressings

Suture—Type of Suture, Needle (if applicable), and Anticipated Tissue Usage

Pharmaceuticals

Miscellaneous

14. Operative preparation:

15. What type of anesthesia will likely be used? Why?

16. List any special anesthesia equipment that may be needed.

17. Patient position during the procedure:

18. What supplies will be necessary for positioning?

____

____

____

____

____

19. What type of shave/skin preparation will be necessary (if any)? ____

____

____

____

____

____

20. Define the anatomic perimeters of the prep.

____

____

____

____

____

____

21. List the order in which the drapes will be applied, and describe any specific variations.

____

____

____

____

____

____

____

22. List any practical considerations.

____

____

____

____

____

____

____

23. List the procedural steps, and describe the preparatory and supportive actions of the STSR during each step (use additional space if necessary).

Operative Procedure	Technical Considerations
1.	•
	•
2.	•
	•
3.	•
	•
4.	•
	•
5.	•
	•

(continues)

Operative Procedure *(continued)*	**Technical Considerations** *(continued)*
6.	•
	•
7.	•
	•
8.	•
	•
9.	•
	•
10.	•
	•

24. What is the postoperative diagnosis? ______________

25. Describe the immediate postoperative care.

26. What is the patient's long-term prognosis?

27. What are the possible complications? ______________

28. Comments or questions: ______________

29. What is the most valuable information you obtained from preparing this surgical procedure case study?

Case Studies

☐ CASE STUDY 1

Lin Su is a 21-year-old female college student. She was admitted to the college's health center for right lower quadrant pain, nausea, and low-grade fever. She was diagnosed with acute appendicitis, and surgery was scheduled.

1. What causes appendicitis?

2. What are the signs and symptoms of appendicitis?

3. Describe a McBurney's incision.

4. What is the primary difference between a McBurney's and a Rockey-Davis incision?

☐

☐ CASE STUDY 2

Jon and Linda are both 41-year-old computer programmers. They are in the preoperative holding area. Each is scheduled for a hernia repair in the groin area.

1. What are the chances that Jon's hernia is a femoral hernia?

2. Jon's hernia is said to be incarcerated. What does this mean?

3. If Linda has a femoral hernia, the hernia exists below what anatomical marker?

4. Describe Hesselbach's triangle.

5. Jon's hernia was described in the postoperative report as a direct hernia. Is it probable that the hernia was congenital in nature?

☐

CHAPTER 15

Obstetric and Gynecologic Surgery

OBJECTIVES

After studying this chapter, the reader should be able to:

A 1. Discuss the relevant anatomy and physiology of the female reproductive system.

P 2. Describe the pathology of the female reproductive system that prompts surgical intervention and the related terminology.

3. Discuss any special preoperative obstetric and gynecologic diagnostic procedures/tests.

O 4. Discuss any special preoperative preparation procedures related to obstetric/gynecologic procedures.

5. Identify the names and uses of obstetric and gynecologic instruments, supplies, and drugs.

6. Identify the names and uses of special equipment related to obstetric/gynecologic surgery.

7. Discuss the intraoperative preparation of the patient undergoing an obstetric or gynecologic procedure.

8. Define and give an overview of the obstetric/gynecologic procedure.

9. Discuss the purpose and expected outcomes of the obstetric/gynecologic procedure.

10. Discuss the immediate postoperative care and possible complications of the obstetric/gynecologic procedure.

S 11. Discuss any specific variations related to the preoperative, intraoperative, and postoperative care of the obstetric/gynecologic patient.

Select Key Terms

Define the following:

1. adnexa ______________________________

2. bony pelvis ______________________________

3. breech ______________________________

4. cesarean section ______________________________

5. corpus luteum ______________________________

6. CPD ______________________________

7. curettage ______________________________

8. delivery forceps ______________________________

9. DUB ______________________________

10. dystocia ______________________________

11. episiotomy ______________________________

12. exenteration ______________________________

13. fimbria ______________________________

14. fistula ______________________________

15. gravida ______________________________

16. LEEP ______________________________

17. ligament ______________________________

18. marsupialization ______________________________

19. myoma ______________________________

20. occiput anterior ______________________________

21. parity ______________________________

22. perineum ______________________________

23. Pfannenstiel ______________________________

24. vestibule ______________________________

Exercise A – Anatomy

1. Identify the structures of the external female genitalia shown in Figure 15-1.

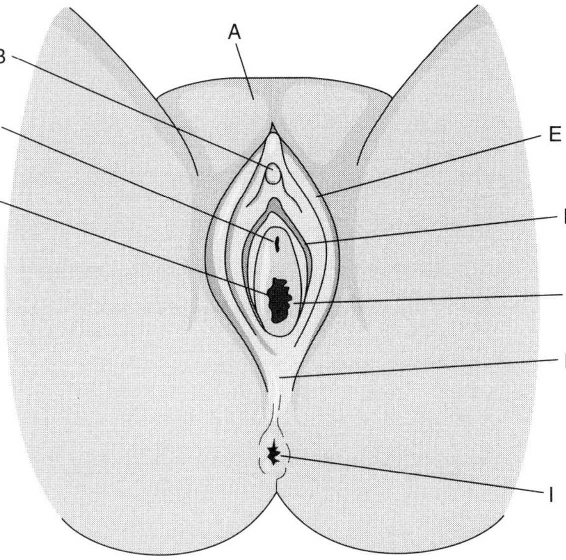

Figure 15-1

A. ____________________

B. ____________________

C. ____________________

D. ____________________

E. ____________________

F. ____________________

G. ____________________

H. ____________________

I. ____________________

2. Identify the structures shown in Figure 15-2.

A. ____________________

B. ____________________

C. ____________________

D. ____________________

E. ____________________

F. ____________________

G. ____________________

H. ____________________

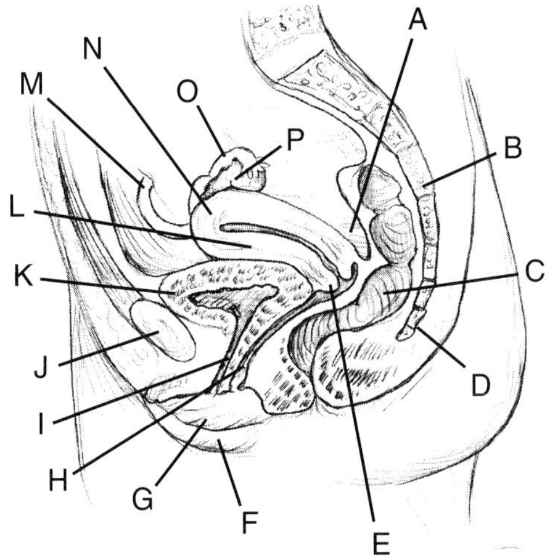

Figure 15-2

I. ____________________

J. ____________________

K. ____________________

L. ____________________

M. ____________________

N. ____________________

O. ____________________

P. ____________________

3. Identify the structures of the female reproductive system shown in Figure 15-3.

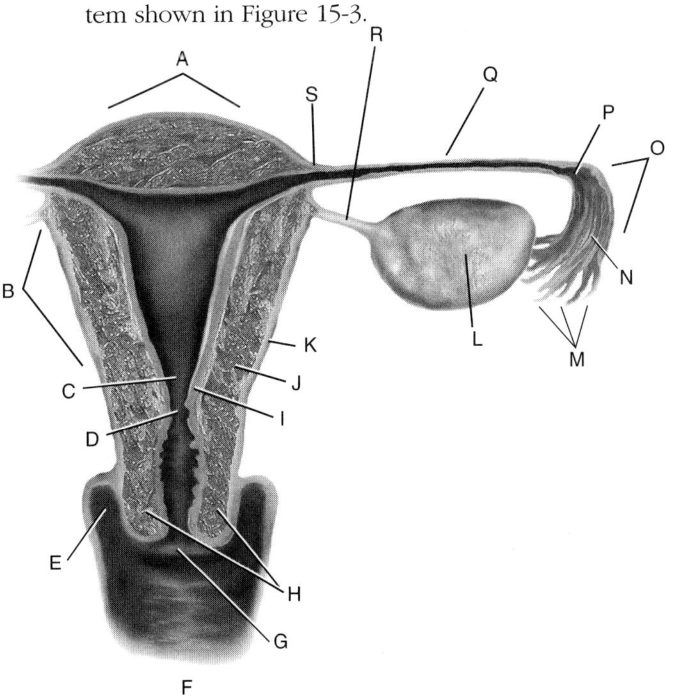

Figure 15-3

A. ______________________

B. ______________________

C. ______________________

D. ______________________

E. ______________________

F. ______________________

G. ______________________

H. ______________________

I. ______________________

J. ______________________

K. ______________________

L. ______________________

M. ______________________

N. ______________________

O. ______________________

P. ______________________

Q. ______________________

R. ______________________

S. ______________________

4. What is the fornix? ______________________

____

____

5. Describe the locations of the internal and external cervical os. ______________________

____

____

6. List the three layers of the uterine wall.

A. ______________________

B. ______________________

C. ______________________

7. Where are the Bartholin's glands located? What is their function? ______________________

____

____

8. List the structures contained within the broad ligament.

A. ______________________

B. ______________________

C. ______________________

D. ______________________

E. ______________________

F. ______________________

9. What are the other two names for the fallopian tubes?

____

____

____

10. Describe the location of the ovaries. ______________________

____

____

11. Name the two hormones from the anterior pituitary that stimulate the ovarian cycle. ______________________

____

____

12. Name the two hormones that are produced by the ovary. ______________________

____

____

13. Name the bones of the pelvic girdle. ______________________

____

____

14. What is the main muscle of the pelvic floor? Name its three components. ______________________

____

A. ______________________

B. ______________________

C. ______________________

15. Branches of which nerve provide sensation to the perineum? ______________________

____

____

Exercise B – Pathology

1. Are Braxton Hicks contractions an indication that delivery of the fetus is imminent? ______

2. Cord blood is collected routinely with every delivery. Why? ______

3. What does "fetal distress" mean? ______

4. What is the most common reason for performing a cesarean section? ______

5. Define *cystocele*, and give two reasons why a cystocele may occur. ______

6. What condition is diagnosed with the use of the Pap smear? ______

7. List the possible sites for ectopic pregnancy.

8. What is meant by the term *incompetent cervix*? What procedure is performed to treat the condition during pregnancy? ______

9. Define *leiomyoma*. ______

10. What are the symptoms of endometriosis? ______

11. Is ultrasound useful in diagnosing a malignancy?

12. What is the most common symptom of uterine cancer? ______

13. List two placental conditions that may necessitate a cesarean section. ______

14. Amenorrhea is the condition of ______.

15. What is a pedunculated lesion? ______

Exercise C – Operation

1. In what position will the patient be placed to accomplish a D&C? In addition to the basic position, which position may be used to enhance the surgeon's view of the anatomy? ______

2. Explain the usefulness of the Trendelenburg position during pelvic surgery. ______

3. Describe the complications that the patient may suffer from an undiagnosed or improperly closed perineal laceration. ______

4. Name two types of suction devices that may be used to clear a neonate's airway. ______________________

____

____

5. What are the advantages to a "classic" approach for a cesarean section? ______________________

____

____

6. Name the three approaches that are available for tubal sterilization.

A. ______________________

B. ______________________

C. ______________________

7. Posterior colporrhaphy is performed to treat which condition? ______________________

____

____

8. What is Lugol's solution used for? ______________________

____

____

9. What are some advantages to LAVH? ______________________

____

____

10. What is the importance of draining the bladder prior to D&C? ______________________

____

____

11. Why is a Foley catheter placed prior to a cesarean section? ______________________

____

____

12. List the structures that will be removed during total pelvic exenteration. ______________________

____

____

13. What safety measures must be implemented when a laser is in use? ______________________

____

____

14. List the drape components that are necessary to drape a patient in the lithotomy position. Describe the draping sequence. ______________________

____

____

15. What structure(s) is/are removed during a TAH? ___

____

____

Exercise D – Specific Variations

Student Name ______________________ Date ____________

Instructor ______________________

Surgical Procedure – Student Case Study Report

The student will be provided with basic patient information (real or simulated) and is expected to complete the following case study.

1. Procedure name: ______________________

2. Definition of procedure: ______________________

3. What is the purpose of the procedure? ______________________

4. What is the expected outcome of the procedure?

5. Patient age: ______________________

6. Gender: ______________________

7. Additional pertinent patient information: ______________________

8. Probable preoperative diagnosis: ______________________

9. How was the diagnosis determined? ______________________

10. Discuss the relevant anatomy. ______________________

11. List the general and procedure-specific equipment that will be needed for the procedure.

12. List the general and procedure-specific instruments that will be needed for the procedure.

______ ______
______ ______
______ ______
______ ______
______ ______
______ ______

13. List the basic and procedure-specific supplies that will be needed for the procedure.

Pack ______

Basin ______

Gloves ______

Blades ______

Drapes ______

______

Drains ______

Dressings ______

______

Suture—Type of Suture, Needle (if applicable), and Anticipated Tissue Usage

______ ______
______ ______
______ ______
______ ______
______ ______
______ ______
______ ______

Pharmaceuticals

______ ______
______ ______
______ ______
______ ______
______ ______

Miscellaneous

______ ______
______ ______
______ ______
______ ______
______ ______
______ ______

14. Operative preparation: ______

______
______
______
______
______
______

15. What type of anesthesia will likely be used? Why?

______
______
______
______
______

16. List any special anesthesia equipment that may be needed. ______

______
______
______
______
______
______

17. Patient position during the procedure: ______

______
______
______
______

18. What supplies will be necessary for positioning?

____

____

____

____

____

19. What type of shave/skin preparation will be necessary (if any)? _______________

____

____

____

____

____

20. Define the anatomic perimeters of the prep.

____

____

____

____

____

____

21. List the order in which the drapes will be applied, and describe any specific variations.

____

____

____

____

____

____

____

22. List any practical considerations.

____

____

____

____

____

____

____

23. List the procedural steps, and describe the preparatory and supportive actions of the STSR during each step (use additional space if necessary).

Operative Procedure	Technical Considerations
1.	•
	•
2.	•
	•
3.	•
	•
4.	•
	•
5.	•
	•

(continues)

Operative Procedure *(continued)*	Technical Considerations *(continued)*
6.	•
	•
7.	•
	•
8.	•
	•
9.	•
	•
10.	•
	•

24. What is the postoperative diagnosis? ____________

25. Describe the immediate postoperative care.

26. What is the patient's long-term prognosis?

27. What are the possible complications? ____________

28. Comments or questions: ____________

29. What is the most valuable information you obtained from preparing this surgical procedure case study?

Case Studies

☐ CASE STUDY 1

Shannon is a 23-year-old primipara who has just been admitted to the labor and delivery unit. She has had a normal pregnancy, and sonograms confirm only one fetus. Her cervix is dilated to 4 cm.

1. How long, on average, would you expect her labor to continue?

2. To what does the term *presentation* refer?

3. To what does the term *position* refer?

4. To what does the term *station* refer?

☐

☐ CASE STUDY 2

Correta has been admitted for a diagnostic laparoscopy for pelvic pain of unknown origin.

1. What equipment will be needed for the procedure?

2. What instruments will be needed for the procedure?

3. In what position will Correta be placed?

4. What are the common complications of laparoscopy?

CHAPTER 16

Ophthalmic Surgery

OBJECTIVES

After studying this chapter, the reader should be able to:

A 1. Discuss the anatomy of the eye.

P 2. Describe the pathology that prompts surgical intervention of the eye and related terminology.

3. Discuss any special preoperative ophthalmic diagnostic procedures/tests.

O 4. Discuss any special preoperative preparation procedures.

5. Identify the names and uses of ophthalmic instruments, supplies, and drugs.

6. Identify the names and uses of special equipment.

7. Discuss the intraoperative preparation of the patient undergoing an ophthalmic procedure.

8. Define and give an overview of the ophthalmic procedure.

9. Discuss the purpose and expected outcomes of the ophthalmic procedures.

10. Discuss the immediate postoperative care and possible complications of the ophthalmic procedures.

S 11. Discuss any specific variations related to the preoperative, intraoperative, and postoperative care of the ophthalmic patient.

Select Key Terms

Define the following:

1. anterior chamber ______
2. BSS ______
3. cataract ______
4. chalazion ______
5. dacryo- ______
6. diathermy ______
7. enucleation ______
8. extracapsular cataract extraction ______
9. extrinsic muscles ______
10. globe ______
11. intracapsular cataract extraction ______
12. iridotomy ______
13. kerato- ______
14. lacrimal ______
15. ocutome ______
16. posterior chamber ______
17. retrobulbar ______
18. strabismus ______
19. trephine ______
20. tunic ______

Exercise A – Anatomy

1. Identify the structures of the eye shown in Figure 16-1.

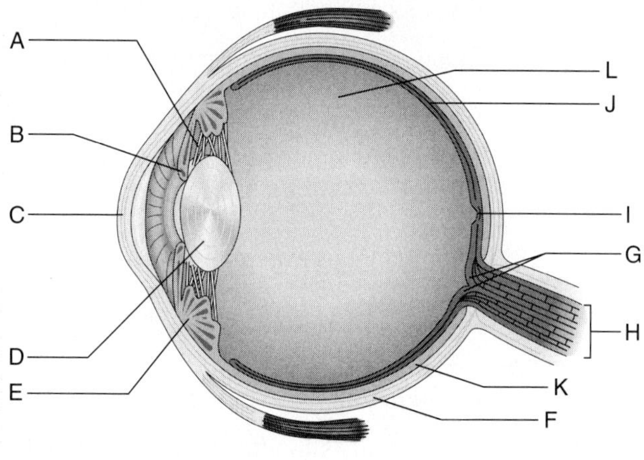

Figure 16-1

A. ______
B. ______
C. ______
D. ______
E. ______
F. ______
G. ______
H. ______
I. ______

J. ______________________________

K. ______________________________

L. ______________________________

2. Identify the nerves of the eye shown in Figure 16-2.

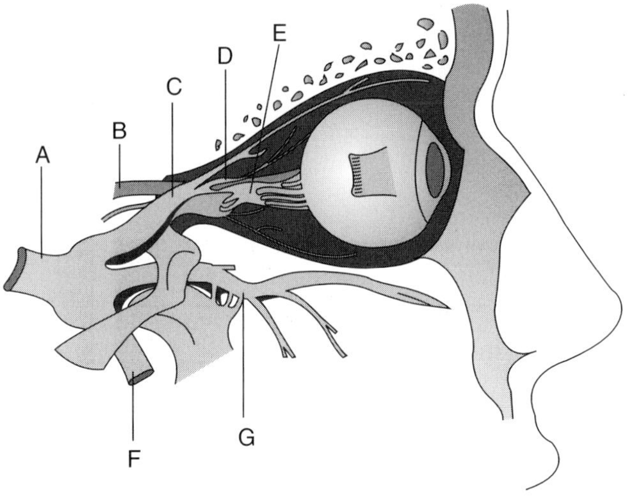

Figure 16-2

A. ______________________________

B. ______________________________

C. ______________________________

D. ______________________________

E. ______________________________

F. ______________________________

G. ______________________________

3. Identify the muscles of the eye shown in Figure 16-3.

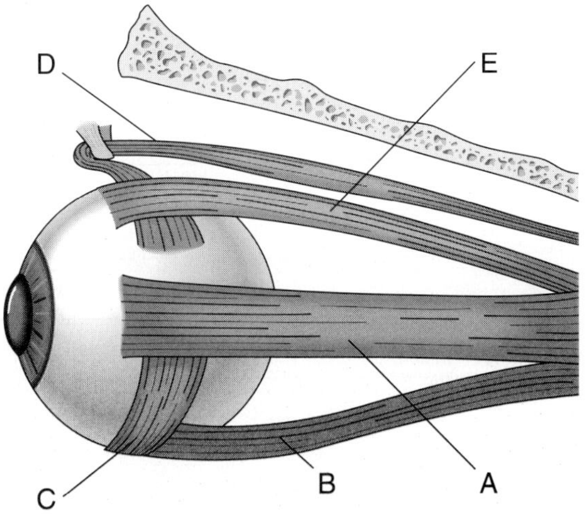

Figure 16-3

A. ______________________________

B. ______________________________

C. ______________________________

D. ______________________________

E. ______________________________

4. Identify the structures of the lacrimal apparatus shown in Figure 16-4.

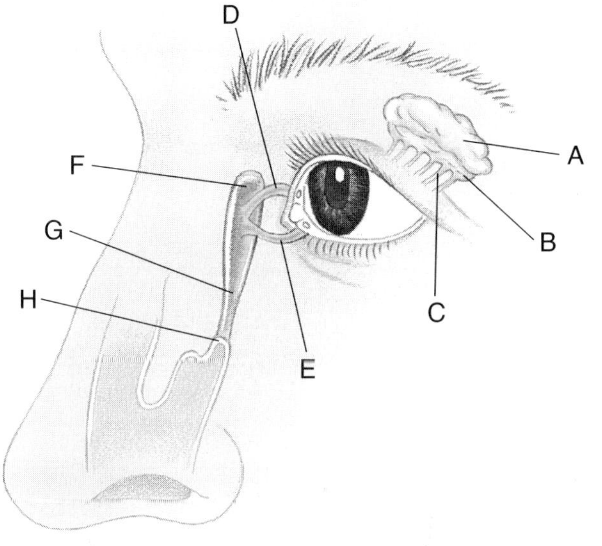

Figure 16-4

A. ______________________________

B. ______________________________

C. ______________________________

D. ______________________________

E. ______________________________

F. ______________________________

G. ______________________________

H. ______________________________

5. Name the three tunics of the eye.

A. ______________________________

B. ______________________________

C. ______________________________

6. Name the two intrinsic muscles of the eye.

A. ____________________

B. ____________________

7. Name the bones that form the orbit.

A. ____________________

B. ____________________

C. ____________________

D. ____________________

E. ____________________

F. ____________________

G. ____________________

8. Name the six extrinsic muscles of the eye and the primary function of each.

A. ____________________

B. ____________________

C. ____________________

D. ____________________

E. ____________________

F. ____________________

9. What are the four tissue layers that make up the cornea?

A. ____________________

B. ____________________

C. ____________________

D. ____________________

10. ________________ humor fills the posterior chamber of the eye.

11. Briefly explain the process of accommodation.

____

____

____

____

12. Describe the location of the crystalline lens.

____

____

____

____

13. List the refractive media of the eye.

A. ____________________

B. ____________________

C. ____________________

D. ____________________

14. What is the function of the iris? ____________________

____

____

____

____

15. Describe the functions of the rods and the cones.

____

____

____

____

Exercise B – Pathology

1. Give three reasons for cataract formation.

A. ____________________

B. ____________________

C. ____________________

2. Why is a cataract considered a condition rather than a disease? ____________________

____

____

____

____

3. Describe what happens when a retinal detachment occurs. ______________________________

____

____

____

____

4. Explain why a patient may see "spots" or "flashes of light" with the development of a retinal detachment.

____

____

____

____

5. What is a chalazion? ______________________________

____

____

____

____

6. Explain the difference between comitant and incomitant strabismus. ______________________________

____

____

____

____

7. List four causes of corneal clouding.

A. ______________________________

B. ______________________________

C. ______________________________

D. ______________________________

8. Name and describe the visual defect shown in Figure 16-5.

____

____

____

____

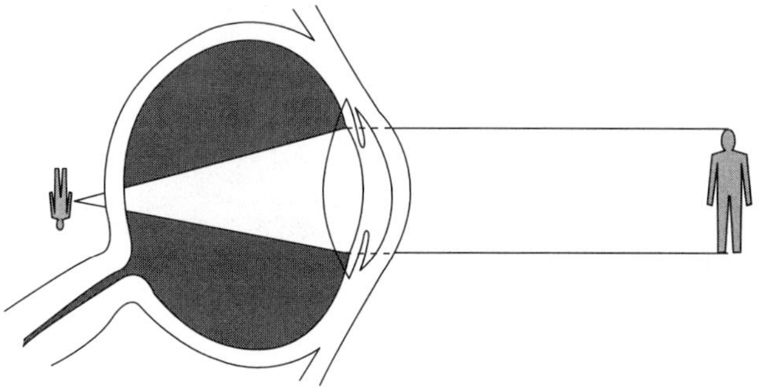

Figure 16-5

9. Name and describe the visual defect shown in Figure 16-6.

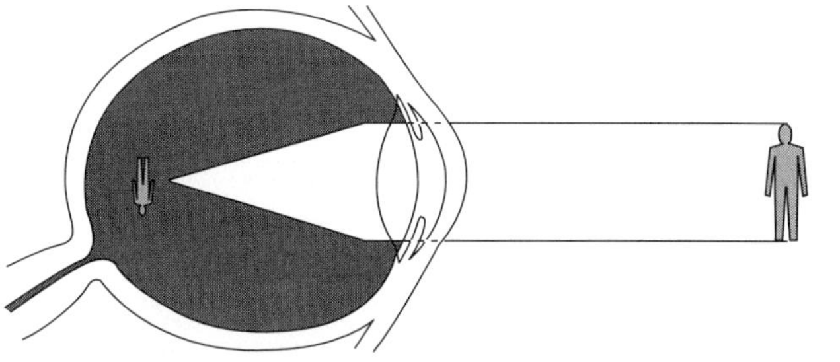

Figure 16-6

____

____

____

____

____

10. Name and describe the visual defect shown in Figure 16-7.

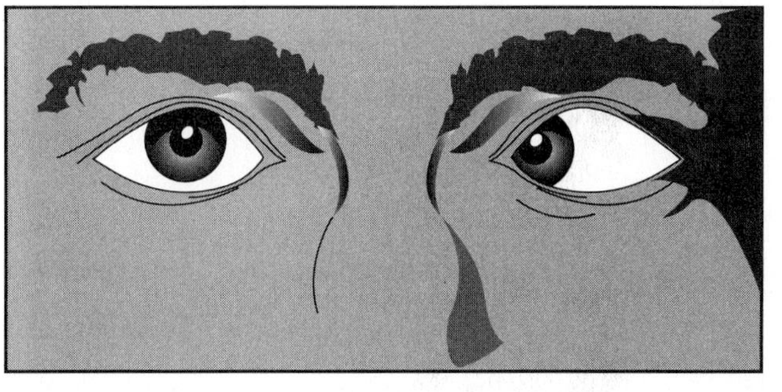

Figure 16-7

____

____

____

____

11. Name and describe the visual defect shown in Figure 16-8.

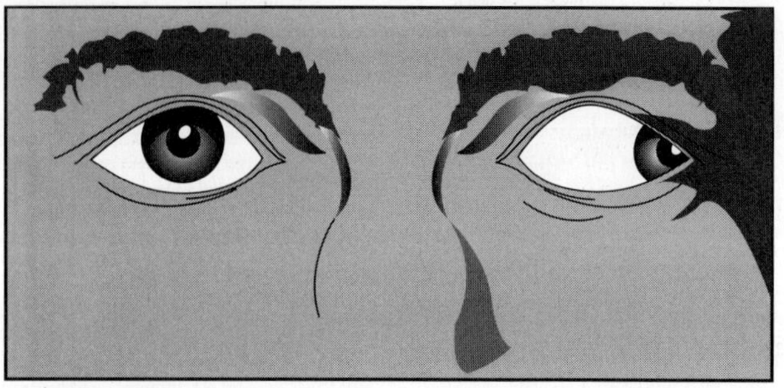

Figure 16-8

12. What condition is characterized by excess pressure of the aqueous humor?

13. What is an epiretinal membrane?

14. List three indications for enucleation.

A.

B.

C.

15. What visual deficit will occur in a person who lacks cones in the retina?

Exercise C – Operation

1. How is intraocular pressure measured from within the sterile field?

2. What procedure is performed to open the blocked tear ducts of an infant?

3. List three methods for cataract extraction.

A.

B.

C.

4. What is a diathermy apparatus used to accomplish?

5. How is cryotherapy used to treat retinal detachment?

6. Recession/resection is used for correcting what condition of the eye?

7. What type of instrument is a trephine? In eye surgery, what is it used for? ______________________

____

____

____

____

8. What is the purpose of inserting a scleral buckle to treat retinal detachment? ______________________

____

____

____

____

9. List four complications that may arise following a scleral buckle procedure.

A. ______________________

B. ______________________

C. ______________________

D. ______________________

10. The topical anesthetic cocaine is often used to prepare the nose for dacryocystorhinostomy, even if a general anesthetic is planned. Why?

____

____

____

____

11. What is the main advantage of evisceration of the eye over enucleation?

____

____

____

____

12. What is sodium hyaluronate used for?

____

____

____

13. List the drapes necessary for surgery to expose the eye, and their order of application.

____

____

____

____

14. What is the purpose of applying fluorescein to the cornea? What tool must be used in conjunction with fluorescein?

____

____

____

____

15. What is the main advantage of phacoemulsification over traditional extracapsular cataract extraction?

____

____

____

____

Exercise D – Specific Variations

Student Name ______________________________ Date ______________

Instructor ______________________________

Surgical Procedure – Student Case Study Report

The student will be provided with basic patient information (real or simulated) and is expected to complete the following case study.

1. Procedure name: ______________________________

2. Definition of procedure: ______________________________

3. What is the purpose of the procedure? ______________________________

4. What is the expected outcome of the procedure?

5. Patient age: ______________________________

6. Gender: ______________________________

7. Additional pertinent patient information: ______________________________

8. Probable preoperative diagnosis: ______________________________

9. How was the diagnosis determined? ______________________________

10. Discuss the relevant anatomy. ______________________________

11. List the general and procedure-specific equipment that will be needed for the procedure.

12. List the general and procedure-specific instruments that will be needed for the procedure.

13. List the basic and procedure-specific supplies that will be needed for the procedure.

Pack

Basin

Gloves

Blades

Drapes

Drains

Dressings

Suture—Type of Suture, Needle (if applicable), and Anticipated Tissue Usage

Pharmaceuticals

Miscellaneous

14. Operative preparation:

15. What type of anesthesia will likely be used? Why?

16. List any special anesthesia equipment that may be needed.

17. Patient position during the procedure:

18. What supplies will be necessary for positioning?

___

___

___

___

___

19. What type of shave/skin preparation will be necessary (if any)? ___

___

___

___

___

___

20. Define the anatomic perimeters of the prep.

___

___

___

___

___

___

21. List the order in which the drapes will be applied, and describe any specific variations.

___

___

___

___

___

___

___

22. List any practical considerations.

___

___

___

___

___

___

___

23. List the procedural steps, and describe the preparatory and supportive actions of the STSR during each step (use additional space if necessary).

Operative Procedure	Technical Considerations
1.	•
	•
2.	•
	•
3.	•
	•
4.	•
	•
5.	•
	•

Operative Procedure *(continued)*	**Technical Considerations** *(continued)*
6.	•
	•
7.	•
	•
8.	•
	•
9.	•
	•
10.	•
	•

24. What is the postoperative diagnosis?

25. Describe the immediate postoperative care.

26. What is the patient's long-term prognosis?

27. What are the possible complications?

28. Comments or questions.

29. What is the most valuable information you obtained from preparing this surgical procedure case study?

Case Studies

CASE STUDY 1

Susan is admitted to the hospital for eye surgery. She was diagnosed in childhood with diabetes and is now 50 years old. Susan also has been diagnosed with retinopathy, a frequent occurrence in diabetic patients. Her vision has been deteriorating over the last several years. She has recently suffered a vitreous hemorrhage due to neovascularization of the eye, which is common in diabetic patients.

1. What procedure will be performed to resolve the problem?

2. Briefly describe the procedure, and explain how Susan will benefit.

3. What are the two possible approaches the surgeon may use to enter the eye? Which is preferred?

4. What piece of equipment is crucial to a vitrectomy?

5. What substance, if any, will be used to replace the vitreous humor?

☐ CASE STUDY 2

Ronald has been having trouble with his stereoscopic vision. His wife says that he appears to have a "lazy eye." The amount of misalignment seems to stay the same no matter which direction his eyes are looking. Ronald has been admitted to the ambulatory care center for surgery.

1. What is the correct term for the condition that Ronald has?

2. Would this condition be considered "comitant" or "incomitant?"

3. What surgical procedure will be performed to correct this condition?

4. In which position will Ronald be placed for this procedure?

5. What are the anatomic boundaries for the prep?

☐

Otorhinolaryngologic Surgery

CHAPTER 17

OBJECTIVES

After studying this chapter, the reader should be able to:

A 1. Discuss the relevant anatomy of the ear, nose, and upper aerodigestive tract.

P 2. Describe the pathology that prompts otorhinolaryngologic surgical intervention and the related terminology.

3. Discuss any special preoperative otorhinolaryngologic diagnostic procedures/tests.

O 4. Discuss any special otorhinolaryngologic preoperative preparation procedures.

5. Identify the names and uses of otorhinolaryngologic instruments, supplies, and drugs.

6. Identify the names and uses of special otorhinolaryngologic equipment.

7. Discuss the intraoperative preparation of the patient undergoing an otorhinolaryngologic procedure.

8. Define and give an overview of the otorhinolaryngologic procedures.

9. Discuss the purpose and expected outcomes of the otorhinolaryngologic procedures.

10. Discuss the immediate postoperative care and possible complications of the otorhinolaryngologic procedures.

S 11. Discuss any specific variations related to the preoperative, intraoperative, and postoperative care of the otorhinolaryngologic patient.

Select Key Terms

Define the following:

1. aerodigestive tract ______________________________
2. apnea ______________________________
3. carina ______________________________
4. cholesteatoma ______________________________
5. congenital ______________________________
6. dynamic equilibrium ______________________________
7. epiglottis ______________________________
8. epistaxis ______________________________
9. Gelfoam ______________________________
10. glottis ______________________________
11. hydrops ______________________________
12. hypertrophy ______________________________
13. laryngo- ______________________________
14. myringo- ______________________________
15. olfaction ______________________________
16. oropharynx ______________________________
17. oto- ______________________________
18. pharyngotympanic tube ______________________________
19. polyp ______________________________
20. polysomnography ______________________________
21. rhino- ______________________________
22. -sclerosis ______________________________
23. SMR ______________________________
24. T&A ______________________________
25. UPPP ______________________________

Exercise A – Anatomy

1. Identify the structures of the ear shown in Figure 17-1.

A. ____________ B. ____________

C. ____________ D. ____________

E. ____________ F. ____________

G. ____________ H. ____________

2. Identify the structures of the upper aerodigestive tract shown in Figure 17-2.

A. ____________ B. ____________

C. ____________ D. ____________

E. ____________ F. ____________

G. ____________ H. ____________

I. ____________ J. ____________

K. ____________ L. ____________

M. ____________ N. ____________

O. ____________ P. ____________

Q. ____________

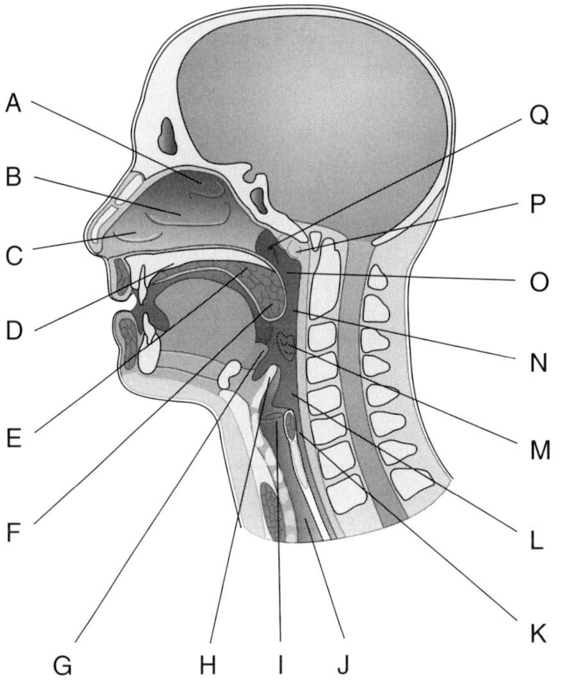

Figure 17-2

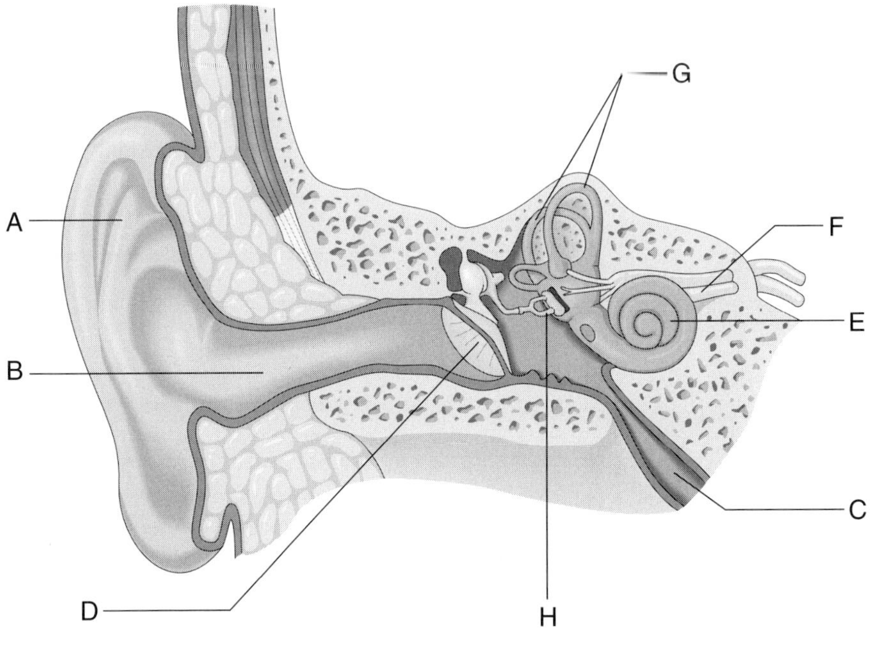

Figure 17-1

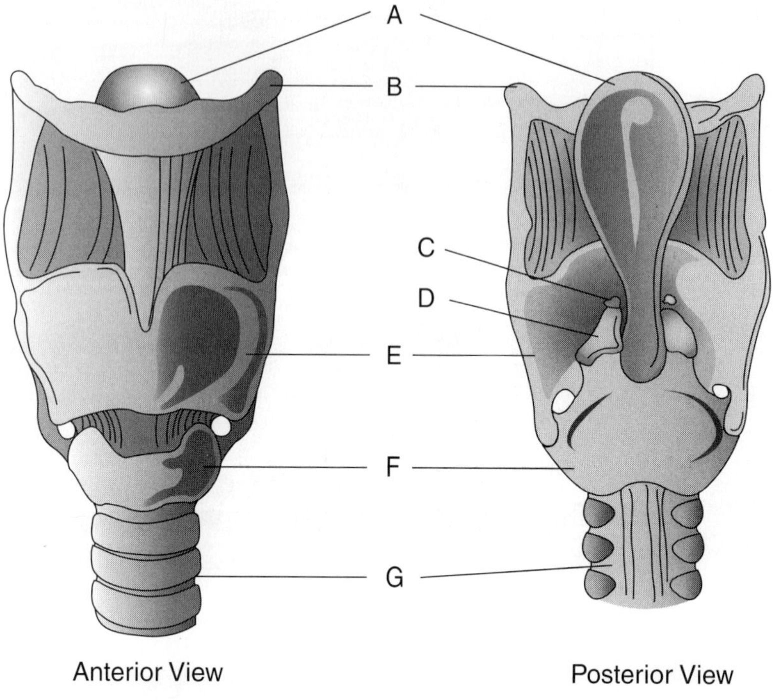

Figure 17-3

3. Identify the structures shown in Figure 17-3.

A. ______

B. ______

C. ______

D. ______

E. ______

F. ______

G. ______

4. List two functions of the nose.

A. ______

______

B. ______

______

5. Which bone houses the mastoid sinus? ______

______

______

______

6. Name the three sections of the pharynx. ______

A. ______

B. ______

C. ______

7. Which of the tonsils are removed during a tonsillectomy? ______

______

______

______

______

8. Name the four pairs of paranasal sinuses, and give their locations.

A. ______

B. ______

C. ______

D. ______

9. How many layers comprise the tympanic membrane, and what is the composition of each layer?

10. Where would you find the umbo and cone of light, and what are they?

11. Provide the scientific and common names for the ossicles in their proper sequence, moving from lateral to medial.

12. How many nasal bones does each individual normally have, and what is their function?

13. What are nasal conchae? Describe their function.

14. What is the main source of arterial blood to the nose, and from which vessel is it derived?

15. Where are the adenoids located?

Exercise B – Pathology

1. Can tonsillitis affect the palatine tonsils?

2. Which nerve is affected in a patient with sensorineural deafness?

3. What is the cause of hypertrophied turbinates?

4. What is the cause of obstructive sleep apnea?

5. What is the most common cause of otitis media?

6. What causes the nasal septum to deviate from the midline? ______________________

7. Where is a Zenker's diverticulum located, and which diagnostic exam will be helpful in determining the diagnosis? ______________________

8. List the symptoms of Ménière's syndrome.

9. List several reasons for nasal septal perforation.

10. What is the most frequent cause of epiglottitis?

11. Swimmer's ear is a specific example of what more general condition? ______________________

12. What are some of the causes of nasal obstruction?

13. What is the usual cause of a vocal cord nodule?

14. Define deafness. ______________________

15. What is the origin of a polyp? ______________________

Exercise C – Operation

1. What is the name of the procedure used to remove nasal polyps, and what special instrument may be used to perform the procedure?

2. What is the unique feature of the #12 knife blade?

3. Are any special precautions necessary when using a carbon dioxide laser? If so, what are they?

4. Describe the differences between rhinoplasty and septoplasty.

5. Which tonsils are typically removed during a tonsillectomy?

6. What are the reasons for reversing the operating table during ear surgery?

7. Is sinus endoscopy a diagnostic or a functional procedure? Why?

8. An adult patient undergoing tonsillectomy with local anesthesia will be placed in what position?

9. What source of energy will be needed to operate the rotating drill?

10. What is intranasal antrostomy, and what special instrument may be needed to facilitate the procedure?

11. What is the most common autologous site for securing a graft for myringoplasty?

12. What are the classifications for tympanoplasty, and how are they determined?

13. Where is the incision made to facilitate drainage of the frontal sinus?

14. What is the pillar dissector used for?______________

15. Describe panendoscopy, and list any special equipment that may be required. ______________

Exercise D – Specific Variations

Student Name ______________________ Date ____________

Instructor ______________________

Surgical Procedure – Student Case Study Report

The student will be provided with basic patient information (real or simulated) and is expected to complete the following case study.

1. Procedure name: ____________
2. Definition of procedure: ____________
3. What is the purpose of the procedure? ____________
4. What is the expected outcome of the procedure?
5. Patient age: ____________
6. Gender: ____________
7. Additional pertinent patient information: ____________
8. Probable preoperative diagnosis:
9. How was the diagnosis determined? ____________
10. Discuss the relevant anatomy. ____________
11. List the general and procedure-specific equipment that will be needed for the procedure.

12. List the general and procedure-specific instruments that will be needed for the procedure.

13. List the basic and procedure-specific supplies that will be needed for the procedure.

Pack

Basin

Gloves

Blades

Drapes

Drains

Dressings

Suture—Type of Suture, Needle (if applicable), and Anticipated Tissue Usage

Pharmaceuticals

Miscellaneous

14. Operative preparation:

15. What type of anesthesia will likely be used? Why?

16. List any special anesthesia equipment that may be needed.

17. Patient position during the procedure:

18. What supplies will be necessary for positioning?

____

____

____

____

____

19. What type of shave/skin preparation will be necessary (if any)? ______________________________________

____

____

____

____

____

20. Define the anatomic perimeters of the prep.

____

____

____

____

____

____

21. List the order in which the drapes will be applied, and describe any specific variations.

____

____

____

____

____

____

____

22. List any practical considerations.

____

____

____

____

____

____

____

23. List the procedural steps, and describe the preparatory and supportive actions of the STSR during each step (use additional space if necessary).

Operative Procedure	Technical Considerations
1.	•
	•
2.	•
	•
3.	•
	•
4.	•
	•
5.	•
	•

(continues)

Operative Procedure *(continued)*	Technical Considerations *(continued)*
6.	•
	•
7.	•
	•
8.	•
	•
9.	•
	•
10.	•
	•

24. What is the postoperative diagnosis? ______________

25. Describe the immediate postoperative care.

26. What is the patient's long-term prognosis?

27. What are the possible complications? ______________

28. Comments or questions: ______________

29. What is the most valuable information you obtained from preparing this surgical procedure case study?

Case Studies

☐ CASE STUDY 1

Stan, a 46-year-old male, is about to spend the night in the "sleep lab." After numerous complaints from his wife that his heavy snoring is keeping her awake, Stan visited his primary care physician. Following a complete physical, Stan was diagnosed with hypertension and obesity, and he was referred to an otorhinolaryngologist.

1. What tests will Stan undergo in the "sleep lab?" ____________________

2. What diagnosis do you think that the otorhinolaryngologist is considering? ____________________

3. What are Stan's conservative treatment options? ____________________

4. If Stan's condition eventually requires surgery, which procedure will be performed, and what structures will be removed? ____________________

☐

☐ CASE STUDY 2

Fred, a 4-year-old male, has been placed in respite foster care because of his uncontrollable temper tantrums, which include long bouts of screaming. The foster family noticed that Fred's voice was hoarse and that it did not improve over time. He was seen by an otorhinolaryngologist, who determined that Fred has developed nodules on his vocal cords.

1. Is Fred's condition life-threatening? ______________________________

2. How was Fred's condition diagnosed? ______________________________

3. What action will be necessary to treat Fred's condition? ______________________________

4. If surgery is required, what type of procedure will be necessary, and how will it be accomplished?

5. If surgery is necessary, will the foster parents have the legal authority to sign his operative consent?

☐

CHAPTER 18

Oral and Maxillofacial Surgery

OBJECTIVES

After studying this chapter, the reader should be able to:

A 1. Discuss the anatomy relevant to oral and maxillofacial surgery.

P 2. Describe the pathology that prompts oral and maxillofacial surgery and the related terminology.

3. Discuss any special preoperative diagnostic procedures/tests pertaining to oral and maxillofacial surgery.

O 4. Discuss special preoperative preparation procedures related to oral and maxillofacial surgery.

5. Identify the names and uses of oral and maxillofacial instruments, supplies, and drugs.

6. Identify the names and uses of special equipment used for oral and maxillofacial surgery.

7. Discuss the intraoperative preparation of the patient undergoing an oral or maxillofacial procedure.

8. Define and give an overview of oral and maxillofacial procedures.

9. Discuss the purpose and expected outcomes of oral and maxillofacial procedures.

10. Discuss the immediate postoperative care and possible complications of oral and maxillofacial procedures.

S 11. Discuss any specific variations related to the preoperative, intraoperative, and postoperative care of the oral and maxillofacial surgical patient.

Select Key Terms

Define the following:

1. alveolar process ______________________________
2. arthroscopy ______________________________
3. calvarial ______________________________
4. condyle ______________________________
5. coronal flap ______________________________
6. craniosynostosis ______________________________
7. dentition ______________________________
8. glenoid fossa ______________________________
9. gnath- ______________________________
10. labia ______________________________
11. malar bone ______________________________
12. malocclusion ______________________________
13. maxillofacial ______________________________
14. meniscus ______________________________
15. mouth prop ______________________________
16. orbicular ______________________________
17. osteotomy ______________________________
18. pan- ______________________________
19. ramus ______________________________
20. reduction ______________________________
21. sagittal ______________________________
22. symphysis ______________________________
23. TMJ ______________________________

Exercise A – Anatomy

1. Identify the bones of the anterior skull shown in Figure 18-1.

   A. ____________________

   B. ____________________

   C. ____________________

   D. ____________________

   E. ____________________

   F. ____________________

   G. ____________________

   H. ____________________

2. Identify the structures of the lateral skull shown in Figure 18-2.

   A. ____________________

   B. ____________________

   C. ____________________

   D. ____________________

   E. ____________________

   F. ____________________

   G. ____________________

   H. ____________________

   I. ____________________

   J. ____________________

   K. ____________________

   L. ____________________

   M. ____________________

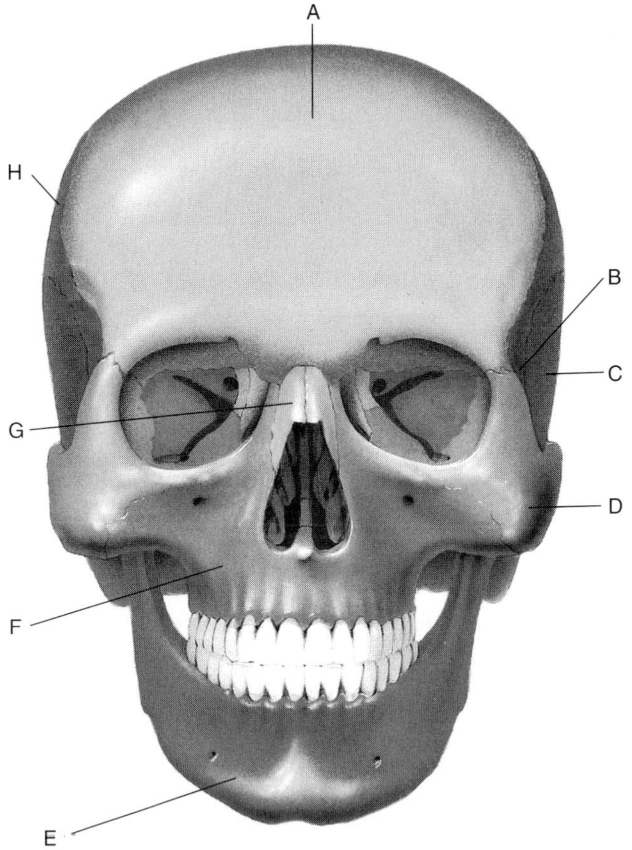

Figure 18-1

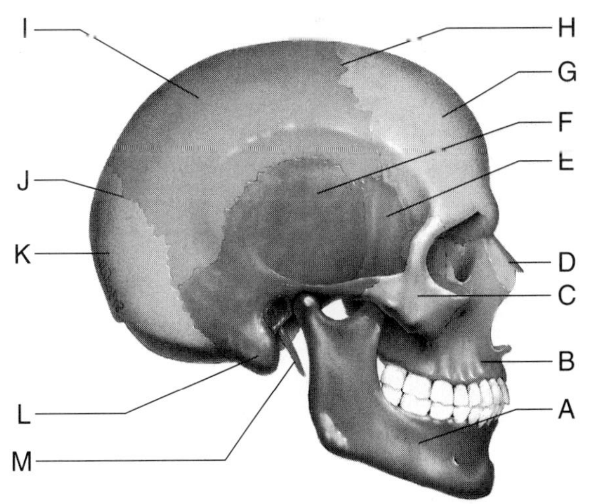

Figure 18-2

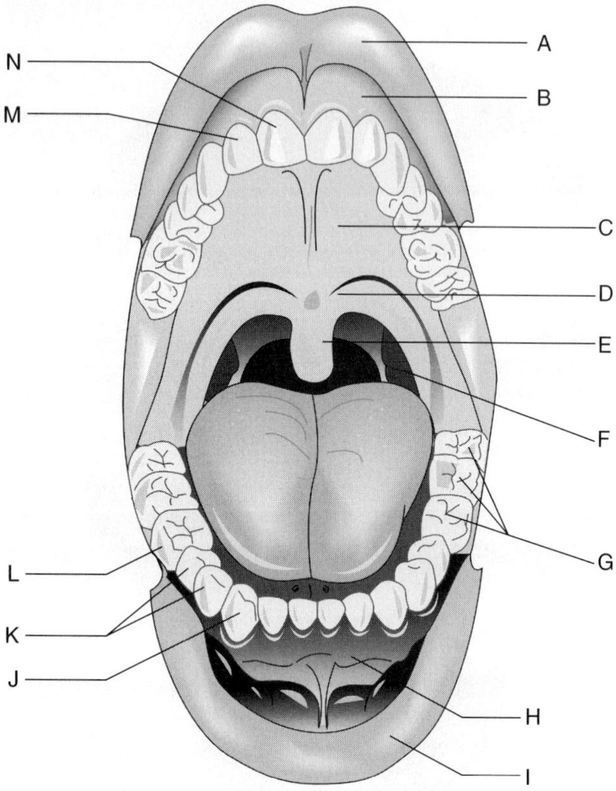

Figure 18-3

3. Identify the structures of the mouth shown in Figure 18-3.

A. ______
B. ______
C. ______
D. ______
E. ______
F. ______
G. ______
H. ______
I. ______
J. ______
K. ______
L. ______
M. ______
N. ______

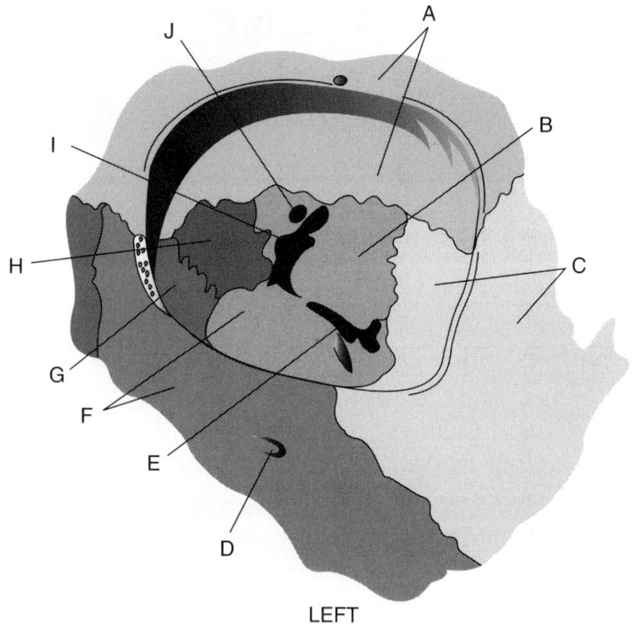

Figure 18-4

4. Identify the structures of the orbit shown in Figure 18-4.

A. ______
B. ______
C. ______
D. ______
E. ______
F. ______
G. ______
H. ______
I. ______
J. ______

5. The anterior portion of the palate is referred to as the ______ palate.

6. What is the location and function of the soft palate?

______
______
______
______

7. The malar bone is also referred to as the _______________ bone.

8. What are the inferior nasal conchae, and what is their function? _______________

9. What is another name for the facial nerve? Which facial muscles are innervated by the facial nerve?

10. Which four muscles control movement of the lower jaw? _______________

11. When does embryologic development of the face occur? _______________

12. Where is the orbicularis oris muscle situated? What is its function? _______________

13. Describe the components and features of the TMJ.

14. What is the ramus of the mandible?

15. What are the two main functions of the orbit?

Exercise B – Pathology

1. What are dental caries, and what is their cause?

2. What is meant by the term *malocclusion*? List two causes.

3. How does Paget's disease affect facial anatomy?

4. Describe a tri-malar fracture. ______________________

5. List the four categories of mandibular fractures.

   A. ______________________

   B. ______________________

   C. ______________________

   D. ______________________

6. What type of midfacial fracture is the most common? ______________________

7. What is laterognathism? List two causes. ______________________

   A. ______________________

   B. ______________________

8. What specific radiographic view is used to detect a fracture of the frontal bone? ______________________

9. Define cerebrospinal rhinorrhea. ______________________

10. List three methods for diagnosing a zygomatic fracture. ______________________

11. List three visual findings that could indicate the presence of a zygomatic fracture.

    A. ______________________

    B. ______________________

    C. ______________________

12. Premature closure of the sutures of the skull is called ______________________.

13. Name and describe the four categories of tooth fractures.

    A. ______________________

    B. ______________________

    C. ______________________

    D. ______________________

14. List two advantages of three-dimensional imaging.

    A. ______________________

    B. ______________________

15. In addition to radiographic studies (including three-dimensional imaging), what other items may be useful to the surgeon during facial reconstruction surgery? ______________________

Exercise C – Operation

1. What is the importance of having the X-rays in the operating room prior to and during the surgical procedure? ______

2. What is accomplished by inserting a mouth prop during certain oral surgical procedures? ______

3. What is the purpose of inserting a throat pack? How is it inserted? ______

4. When is the throat pack removed? Why? ______

5. List two options for sealing an intranasal dural tear.

   A. ______

   B. ______

6. Define ***autogenous,*** and list two possible donor sites for autogenous bone grafts. ______

   A. ______

   B. ______

7. Why is a local anesthetic with epinephrine often injected at the operative site preoperatively when the patient is under general anesthesia? ______

8. Describe the location of a coronal incision. ______

9. List two methods for securing and positioning a soft tissue flap.

   A. ______

   B. ______

10. In what position will the patient be placed for a posterior cranial expansion? ______

11. What type of procedure is performed to treat orthognathia? ______

12. What can be done during lengthy oral procedures to prevent drying and cracking of the lips? ______

13. Why is it important to assure that all metal implants are of the same type?

14. If a bone graft is needed during a procedure in which the patient has a coronal incision, what type of bone will be considered as the first choice? Why?

15. In what situation(s) is arch bar fixation employed?

Exercise D – Specific Variations

Student Name ______________________ Date ______________

Instructor ______________________

Surgical Procedure – Student Case Study Report

The student will be provided with basic patient information (real or simulated) and is expected to complete the following case study.

1. Procedure name: ______________________
2. Definition of procedure: ______________________
3. What is the purpose of the procedure? ______________________
4. What is the expected outcome of the procedure?
5. Patient age: ______________________
6. Gender: ______________________
7. Additional pertinent patient information: ______________________
8. Probable preoperative diagnosis: ______________________
9. How was the diagnosis determined? ______________________
10. Discuss the relevant anatomy. ______________________
11. List the general and procedure-specific equipment that will be needed for the procedure.

12. List the general and procedure-specific instruments that will be needed for the procedure.

13. List the basic and procedure-specific supplies that will be needed for the procedure.

Pack

Basin

Gloves

Blades

Drapes

Drains

Dressings

Suture—Type of Suture, Needle (if applicable), and Anticipated Tissue Usage

Pharmaceuticals

Miscellaneous

14. Operative preparation:

15. What type of anesthesia will likely be used? Why?

16. List any special anesthesia equipment that may be needed.

17. Patient position during the procedure:

18. What supplies will be necessary for positioning?

____

____

____

____

____

19. What type of shave/skin preparation will be necessary (if any)? _______________________________

____

____

____

____

____

20. Define the anatomic perimeters of the prep.

____

____

____

____

____

21. List the order in which the drapes will be applied, and describe any specific variations.

____

____

____

____

____

____

____

22. List any practical considerations.

____

____

____

____

____

____

____

23. List the procedural steps, and describe the preparatory and supportive actions of the STSR during each step (use additional space if necessary).

Operative Procedure	Technical Considerations
1.	•
	•
2.	•
	•
3.	•
	•
4.	•
	•
5.	•
	•

(continues)

Operative Procedure *(continued)*	Technical Considerations *(continued)*
6.	•
	•
7.	•
	•
8.	•
	•
9.	•
	•
10.	•
	•

24. What is the postoperative diagnosis? ______________

____

____

____

____

____

25. Describe the immediate postoperative care.

____

____

____

26. What is the patient's long-term prognosis?

____

____

____

____

____

27. What are the possible complications? ______________

____

____

____

28. Comments or questions: ______________

____

____

____

____

____

____

29. What is the most valuable information you obtained from preparing this surgical procedure case study?

____

____

____

____

____

Case Studies

☐ CASE STUDY 1

Lucricia is a 14-year-old with cerebral palsy and epilepsy. She is scheduled for dental restoration, including gingivectomy for hyperplasia of her gums, under general anesthesia.

1. What procedures may be performed during dental restoration?

2. Why is general anesthesia indicated in Lucricia's case?

3. What is the most likely reason that Lucricia suffers from hyperplasia of her gums that is severe enough to require gingivectomy?

☐ CASE STUDY 2

Roberto experienced a severe blow to his left cheek when he accidentally struck the corner of the wall as he was rushing through a dark hallway during the night, on his way to the bathroom. He is suffering severe pain, and it appears to him that his face no longer has a symmetrical appearance.

1. What type of injury do you suspect that Roberto has incurred? ______________________________

2. What type of examination(s) will be performed by the maxillofacial surgeon to confirm the diagnosis?

3. How will Roberto's problem be corrected? ______________________________

☐

CHAPTER 19

Plastic and Reconstructive Surgery

OBJECTIVES

After studying this chapter, the reader should be able to:

A 1. Discuss the relevant anatomy and physiology of the skin and its underlying tissues.

P 2. Describe the pathology that prompts plastic/reconstructive surgical intervention and the related terminology.

3. Discuss any special preoperative plastic/reconstructive diagnostic procedures/tests.

O 4. Discuss any special preoperative preparation procedures related to plastic/reconstructive surgical procedures.

5. Identify the names and uses of plastic/reconstructive instruments, supplies, and drugs.

6. Identify the names and uses of special equipment related to plastic/reconstructive surgery.

7. Discuss the intraoperative preparation of the patient undergoing a plastic/reconstructive procedure.

8. Define and give an overview of the plastic/reconstructive procedure.

9. Discuss the purpose and expected outcomes of the plastic/reconstructive procedure.

10. Discuss the immediate postoperative care and possible complications of the plastic/reconstructive procedure.

S 11. Discuss any specific variations related to the preoperative, intraoperative, and postoperative care of the plastic/reconstructive patient.

Select Key Terms

Define the following:

1. aesthetic ____________________
2. arthrodesis ____________________
3. augmentation ____________________
4. carpal tunnel ____________________
5. cheiló- ____________________
6. cleft ____________________
7. dermatome ____________________
8. elliptical ____________________
9. ganglion cyst ____________________
10. gynecomastia ____________________
11. integumentary ____________________
12. MPJ ____________________
13. poly- ____________________
14. radial hypoplasia ____________________
15. replantation ____________________
16. rhinoplasty ____________________
17. -schisis ____________________
18. sebum ____________________
19. STSG ____________________
20. syndactyly ____________________
21. synthesis ____________________
22. xenograft ____________________

Exercise A – Anatomy

1. Identify the structures shown in Figure 19-1.

A. ______

B. ______

C. ______

D. ______

E. ______

F. ______

G. ______

H. ______

I. ______

J. ______

K. ______

L. ______

M. ______

N. ______

O. ______

P. ______

Q. ______

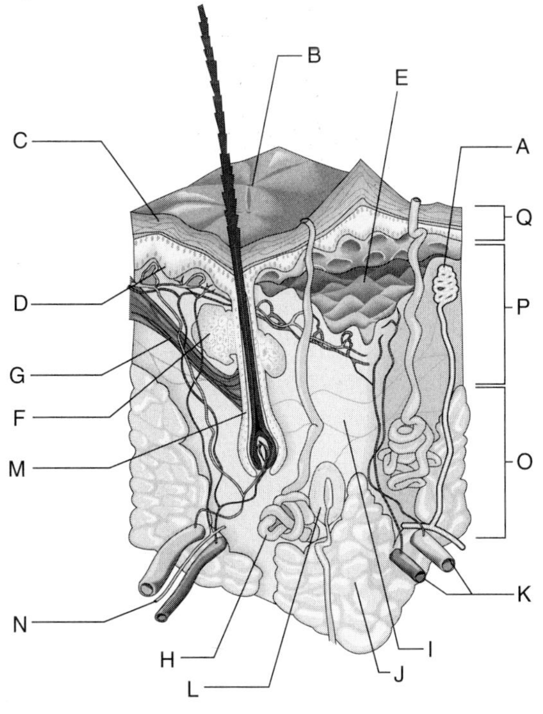

Figure 19-1

2. Identify the bones of the dorsal hand shown in Figure 19-2.

A. ______

B. ______

C. ______

D. ______

E. ______

F. ______

G. ______

H. ______

I. ______

J. ______

K. ______

L. ______

M. ______

N. ______

O. ______

P. ______

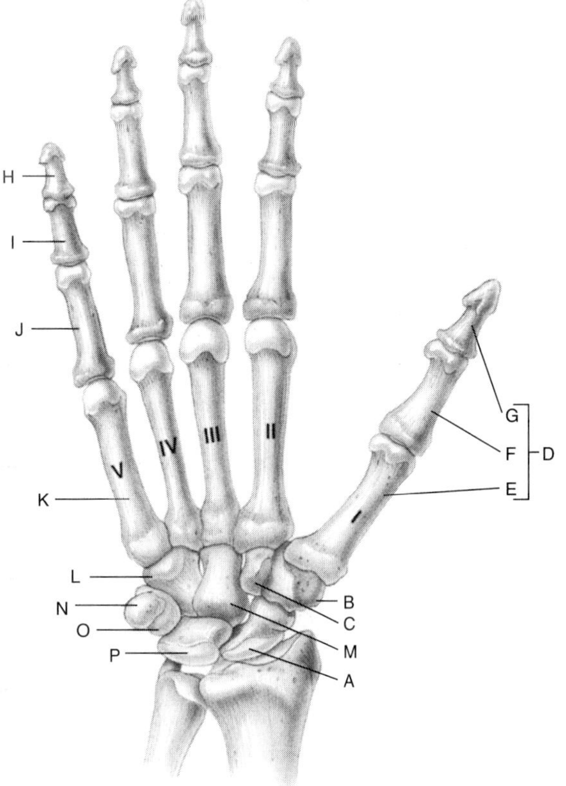

Figure 19-2

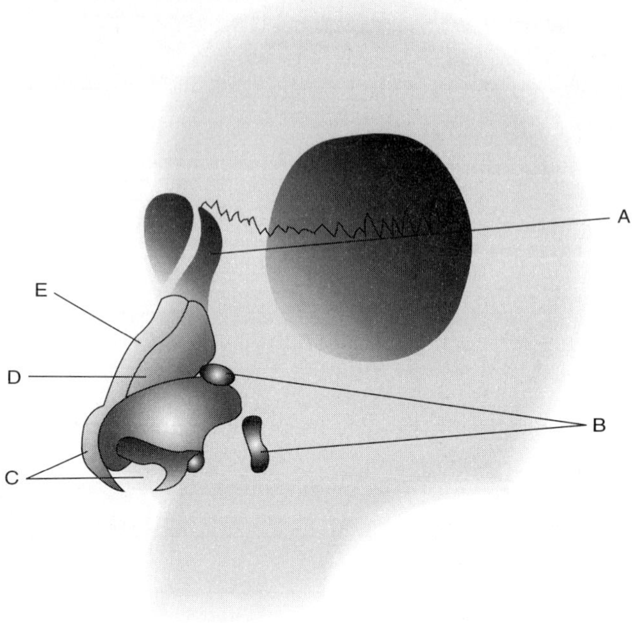

Figure 19-3

3. Identify the nasal structures shown in Figure 19-3.

   A. ______________________

   B. ______________________

   C. ______________________

   D. ______________________

   E. ______________________

4. Identify the structures of the breast shown in Figure 19-4.

   A. ______________________

   B. ______________________

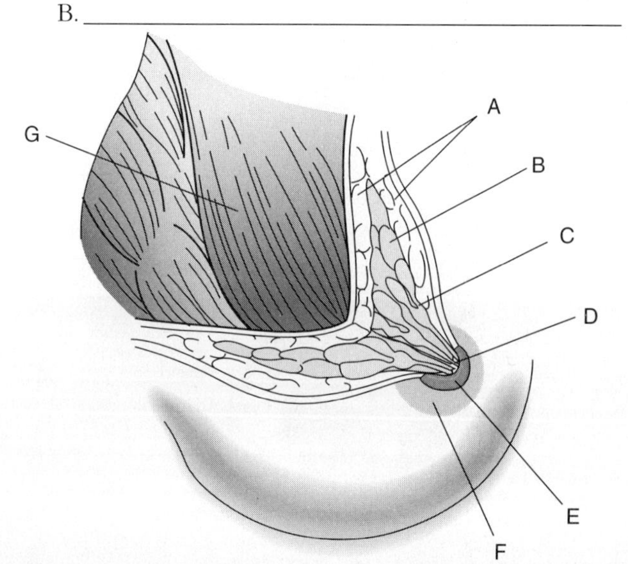

Figure 19-4

   C. ______________________

   D. ______________________

   E. ______________________

   F. ______________________

   G. ______________________

5. Name the two major layers of the integumentary system.

   A. ______________________

   B. ______________________

6. List the major functions of the skin.

   A. ______________________

   B. ______________________

   C. ______________________

   D. ______________________

   E. ______________________

   F. ______________________

   G. ______________________

7. Sweat glands are also known as the _______ glands.

8. Name and briefly describe the three types of sudoriferous glands.

   A. ______________________

   ____

   B. ______________________

   ____

   C. ______________________

9. Name the structures that are contained in the anterior (palmar) compartment of the hand.

   ____

   ____

   ____

   ____

10. Development of the upper limb is complete by the _______ week in utero.

11. Name the five layers of the epidermis in sequence from outermost to innermost layer.

A. ____________

B. ____________

C. ____________

D. ____________

E. ____________

12. Name the three functions of the subcutaneous tissue layer.

A. ____________

B. ____________

C. ____________

13. Name the two divisions of the dermis, and briefly describe them.

A. ____________

B. ____________

14. Name the secretion that is produced in the sebaceous glands. What is the purpose of the secretion? ____________

15. What is the function of the palate? ____________

Exercise B – Pathology

1. Which tissue layer(s) is/are affected by a second-degree burn? ____________

2. Use the Rule of Nines to determine the percentage of the body surface area affected by a third-degree burn of the chest, back, and left arm.

3. Name the bacteria that are the main causative agents of acne vulgaris.

A. ____________

B. ____________

C. ____________

4. Only 20% of cleft deformities are genetic. What is/are the cause(s) of the remaining 80%? ____________

5. What is the most common type of polydactyly?

6. What is a ganglion cyst? ____________

7. What causes the formation of a ganglion cyst?

8. Name three treatment options for a ganglion cyst.

   A. ______________________________

   B. ______________________________

   C. ______________________________

9. What is the cause of ptosis of the eyelid? ______________________________

10. Define neoplasm. Is a neoplasm malignant?

11. Give three examples of common malignant neoplasms of the skin.

    A. ______________________________

    B. ______________________________

    C. ______________________________

12. What is the cause of cheiloschisis and palatoschisis?

13. Name two diseases of the hand that are caused by stenosing tenosynovitis.

    A. ______________________________

    B. ______________________________

14. List two manifestations of palmar fascia contraction (Dupuytren's disease).

    A. ______________________________

    B. ______________________________

15. What is the cause of rheumatoid arthritis? ______________________________

Exercise C – Operation

1. Describe the difference between nasal and rhinoplasty instrumentation. ______________________________

2. What is the purpose/function of a dermatome?

3. List two possible power sources for the oscillating-blade-type dermatome.

   A. ______________________________

   B. ______________________________

4. What is the purpose of a mesh graft device?

5. What is the purpose of a tacking suture? ______________________________

6. What is the advantage of tumescent liposuction over the traditional method? ______________________

7. What is the common name for the umbilical template used during abdominoplasty? What is its purpose?

8. How is sterile mineral oil used during procurement of a STSG? ______________________

9. How is the recipient site prepared prior to placement of a STSG? Why? ______________________

10. Why is palatoplasty considered a clean, rather than sterile, procedure? ______________________

11. What anatomic area is prepped prior to draping for hand surgery? ______________________

12. Why is the extremity wrapped with an Esmarch bandage prior to tourniquet inflation? ______________________

13. Provide two indications for joint replacement in the hand.

A. ______________________

B. ______________________

14. Replantation of a digit begins with the attachment of which structure(s)? ______________________

15. List four incision options that are used to achieve augmentation mammoplasty by producing a minimal or completely hidden scar.

A. ______________________

B. ______________________

C. ______________________

D. ______________________

Exercise D – Specific Variations

Student Name ______________________ Date ____________

Instructor ______________________

Surgical Procedure – Student Case Study Report

The student will be provided with basic patient information (real or simulated) and is expected to complete the following case study.

1. Procedure name: ______________________
2. Definition of procedure: ______________________
3. What is the purpose of the procedure? ______________________
4. What is the expected outcome of the procedure?
5. Patient age: ______________________
6. Gender: ______________________
7. Additional pertinent patient information: ______________________
8. Probable preoperative diagnosis: ______________________
9. How was the diagnosis determined? ______________________
10. Discuss the relevant anatomy. ______________________
11. List the general and procedure-specific equipment that will be needed for the procedure.

12. List the general and procedure-specific instruments that will be needed for the procedure.

______ ______

______ ______

______ ______

______ ______

______ ______

______ ______

13. List the basic and procedure-specific supplies that will be needed for the procedure.

Pack ______

Basin ______

Gloves ______

Blades ______

Drapes ______

______

Drains ______

Dressings ______

______

Suture—Type of Suture, Needle (if applicable), and Anticipated Tissue Usage

______ ______

______ ______

______ ______

______ ______

______ ______

______ ______

Pharmaceuticals

______ ______

______ ______

______ ______

______ ______

______ ______

______ ______

Miscellaneous

______ ______

______ ______

______ ______

______ ______

______ ______

______ ______

14. Operative preparation: ______

______

______

______

______

______

______

15. What type of anesthesia will likely be used? Why?

______

______

______

______

______

16. List any special anesthesia equipment that may be needed. ______

______

______

______

______

______

______

17. Patient position during the procedure: ______

______

______

______

______

18. What supplies will be necessary for positioning?

____

____

____

____

____

19. What type of shave/skin preparation will be necessary (if any)? ______________________________

____

____

____

____

____

20. Define the anatomic perimeters of the prep.

____

____

____

____

____

____

21. List the order in which the drapes will be applied, and describe any specific variations.

____

____

____

____

____

____

____

22. List any practical considerations.

____

____

____

____

____

____

____

23. List the procedural steps, and describe the preparatory and supportive actions of the STSR during each step (use additional space if necessary).

Operative Procedure	Technical Considerations
1.	•
	•
2.	•
	•
3.	•
	•
4.	•
	•
5.	•
	•

Operative Procedure *(continued)*	**Technical Considerations** *(continued)*
6.	•
	•
7.	•
	•
8.	•
	•
9.	•
	•
10.	•
	•

24. What is the postoperative diagnosis? ____________

25. Describe the immediate postoperative care.

26. What is the patient's long-term prognosis?

27. What are the possible complications? ____________

28. Comments or questions: ____________

29. What is the most valuable information you obtained from preparing this surgical procedure case study?

Case Studies

CASE STUDY 1

Three-year-old Bobby accidentally pulled on the tablecloth, causing his mother's scalding coffee to spill on his left neck, shoulder, and chest. It has been determined that Bobby has suffered second- and third-degree burns over 9% of his body. The accident occurred three weeks ago, and Bobby is now scheduled for a STSG.

1. How was the extent of Bobby's injury determined? __________

2. What was the biggest risk that Bobby faced with the third-degree burns? __________

3. What is "STSG," and what special instrument will be required to obtain the graft? __________

4. From which anatomic site is the graft most likely to be procured? __________

☐ CASE STUDY 2

Sven is a 62-year-old dairy farmer. He has been diagnosed with Dupuytren's disease. The disease has progressed to the point where Sven is unable to use his right hand effectively to connect the milking machine to his cows. He has put off surgery as long as possible, but now the inevitable has arrived.

1. What is Dupuytren's disease?

2. Is the condition painful?

3. What procedure will be necessary to treat Sven's condition?

4. Can Sven expect to regain full function and normal appearance?

☐

CHAPTER 20

Genitourinary Surgery

OBJECTIVES

After studying this chapter, the reader should be able to:

A 1. Discuss the relevant anatomy of the genitourinary system.

P 2. Describe the pathology that prompts genitourinary system surgical intervention and the related terminology.

3. Discuss any special preoperative genitourinary diagnostic procedures/tests.

O 4. Discuss any special preoperative genitourinary preparation procedures.

5. Identify the names and uses of genitourinary instruments, supplies, and drugs.
6. Identify the names and uses of special genitourinary equipment.
7. Discuss the intraoperative preparation of the patient undergoing the genitourinary procedure.
8. Define and give an overview of the genitourinary procedure.
9. Discuss the purpose and expected outcomes of the genitourinary procedure.
10. Discuss the immediate postoperative care and possible complications of the genitourinary procedure.

S 11. Discuss any specific variations related to the preoperative, intraoperative, and postoperative care of the genitourinary patient.

Select Key Terms

Define the following:

1. ACTH
2. afferent
3. calculi
4. conduit
5. cortex
6. ESWL
7. focal point
8. Gerota's fascia
9. Gibson incision
10. hilum
11. hirsutism
12. hypertrophy
13. hypospadias
14. incontinence
15. intravenous urogram (IVU)
16. medulla
17. prepuce
18. retroperitoneal
19. stoma
20. suprarenal glands
21. torsion
22. TURP
23. UTI
24. vesical trigone

Exercise A – Anatomy

1. Identify the structures shown in Figure 20-1.

   A. ______________________

   B. ______________________

   C. ______________________

   D. ______________________

   E. ______________________

   F. ______________________

   G. ______________________

   H. ______________________

   I. ______________________

   J. ______________________

   K. ______________________

   L. ______________________

   M. ______________________

   N. ______________________

   O. ______________________

   P. ______________________

   Q. ______________________

   R. ______________________

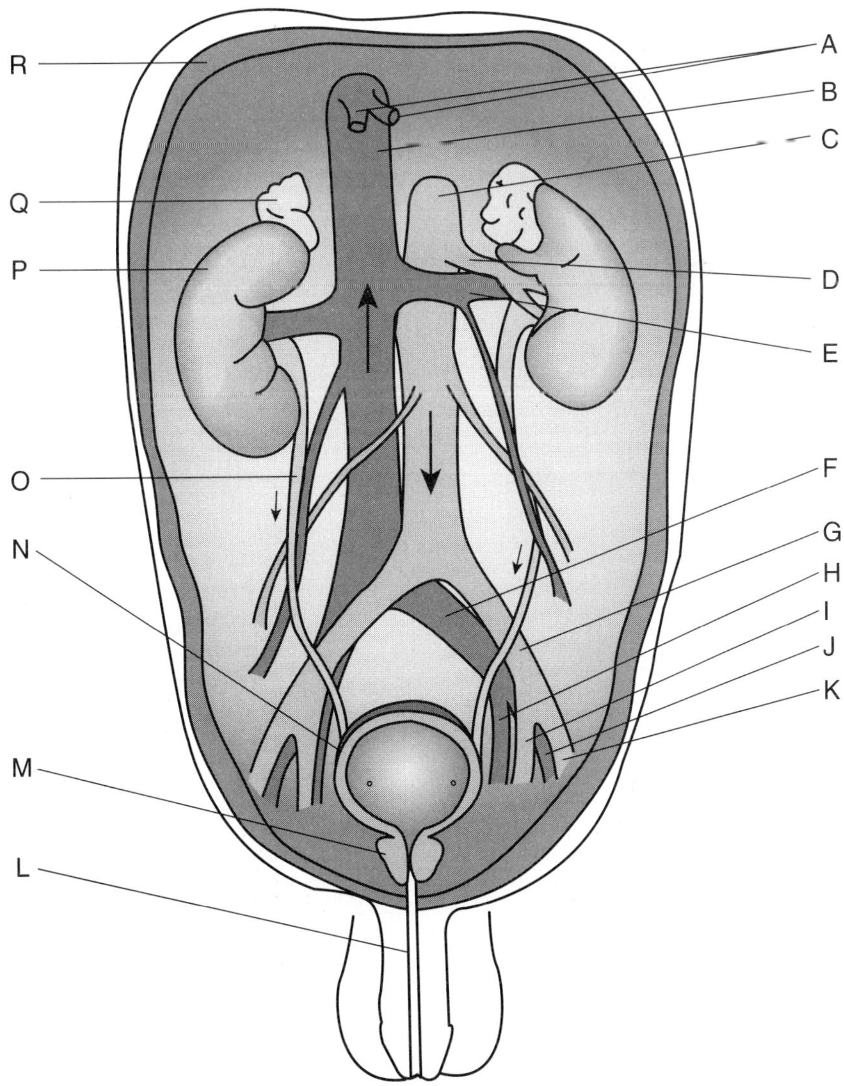

Figure 20-1

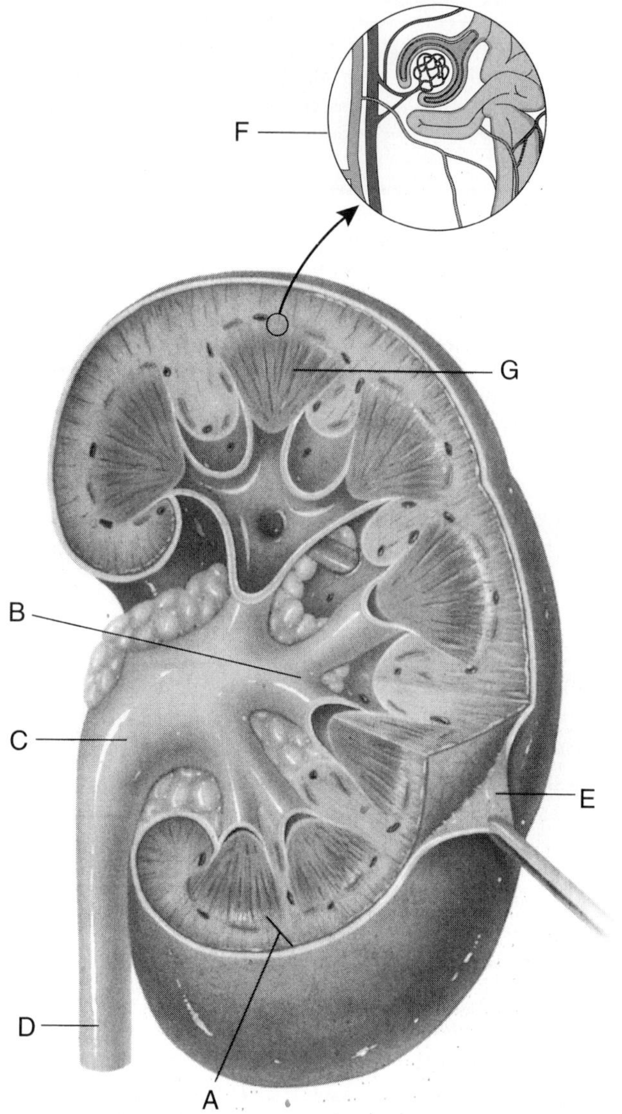

Figure 20-2

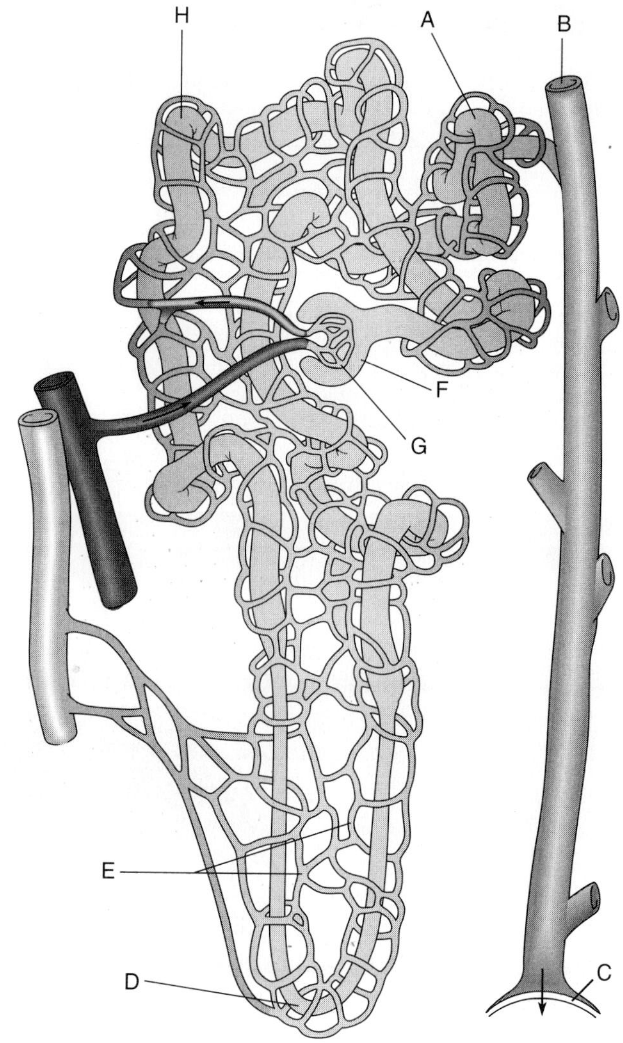

Figure 20-3

2. Identify the structures shown in Figure 20-2.

A. ______

B. ______

C. ______

D. ______

E. ______

F. ______

G. ______

3. Identify the structures shown in Figure 20-3.

A. ______

B. ______

C. ______

D. ______

E. ______

F. ______

G. ______

H. ______

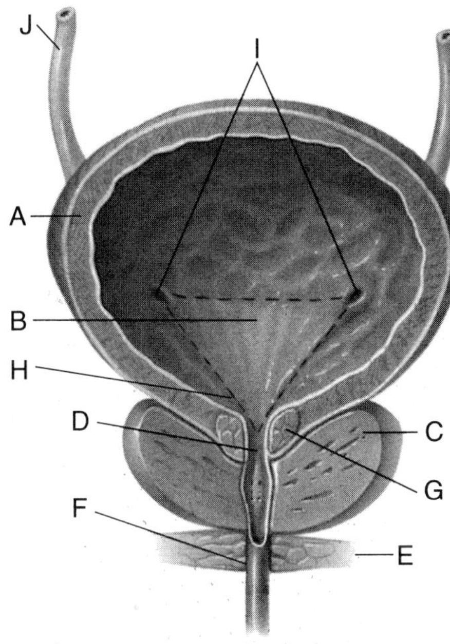

Figure 20-4

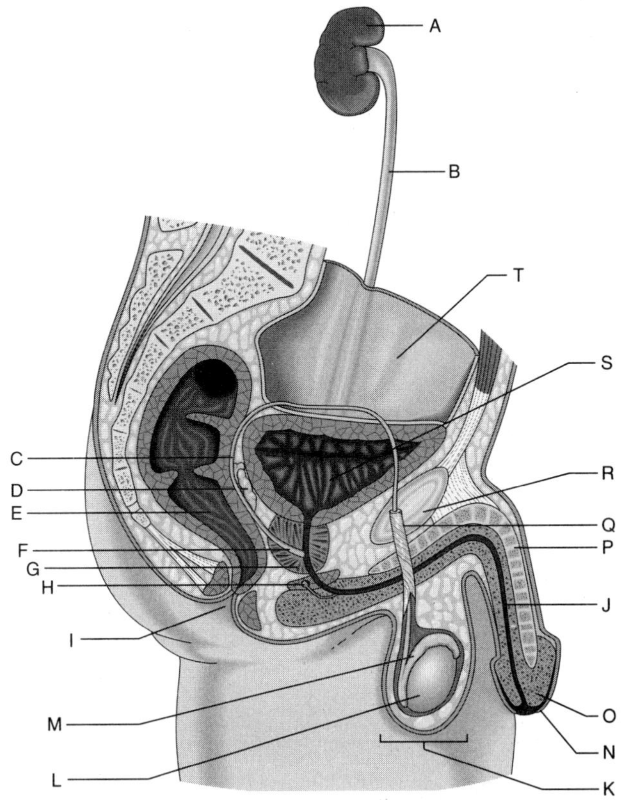

Figure 20-5

4. Identify the structures shown in Figure 20-4.

   A. ______________________

   B. ______________________

   C. ______________________

   D. ______________________

   E. ______________________

   F. ______________________

   G. ______________________

   H. ______________________

   I. ______________________

   J. ______________________

5. Identify the structures shown in Figure 20-5.

   A. ______________________

   B. ______________________

   C. ______________________

   D. ______________________

   E. ______________________

   F. ______________________

   G. ______________________

   H. ______________________

   I. ______________________

   J. ______________________

   K. ______________________

   L. ______________________

   M. ______________________

   N. ______________________

   O. ______________________

   P. ______________________

   Q. ______________________

   R. ______________________

   S. ______________________

   T. ______________________

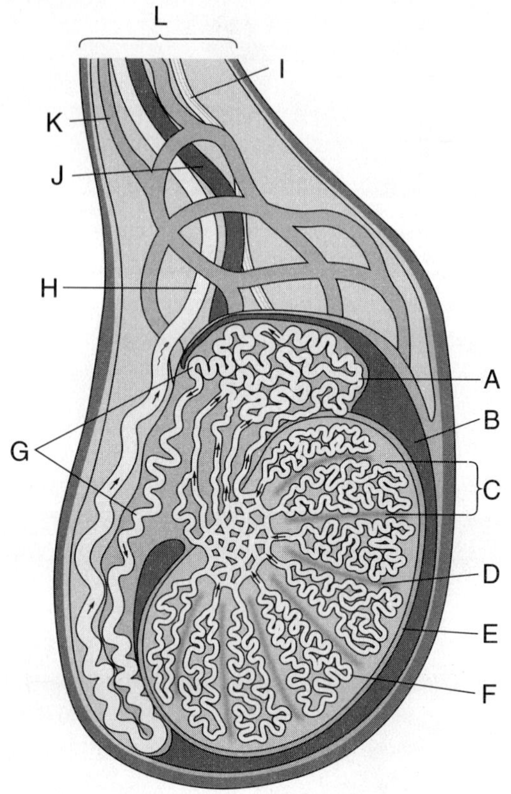

Figure 20-6

6. Identify the structures shown in Figure 20-6.

A. ______________________________

B. ______________________________

C. ______________________________

D. ______________________________

E. ______________________________

F. ______________________________

G. ______________________________

H. ______________________________

I. ______________________________

J. ______________________________

K. ______________________________

L. ______________________________

7. Trace the pathway that sperm cells follow through the ducts of the male reproductive system by placing the following elements in the correct order.

A. ______________ Ductus deferens

B. ______________ Ejaculatory duct

C. ______________ Epididymis

D. ______________ Seminiferous tubules (testis)

E. ______________ Urethra

8. Trace the pathway of fluid from the time it leaves the circulatory system until it leaves the body as urine by placing the following elements in the correct order.

A. ______________ Afferent arteriole

B. ______________ Bladder

C. ______________ Bowman's capsule

D. ______________ Calyx

E. ______________ Collecting tubule

F. ______________ Distal convoluted tubule

G. ______________ Glomerulus

H. ______________ Loop of Henle

I. ______________ Proximal convoluted tubule

J. ______________ Renal artery

K. ______________ Renal pelvis

L. ______________ Ureter

M. ______________ Urethra

9. Name the two portions of the adrenal gland and the function of each.

A. ______________________________

____

B. ______________________________

____

10. Describe the location of the kidneys. ______________

____

____

____

____

11. By what mechanism(s) is/are urine conducted from the kidney to the bladder? ____________________

____

____

____

____

12. What are the anatomic boundaries of the trigone of the bladder? ____________________

____

____

____

____

13. Name the three cavernous structures of the penis.

A. ____________________

B. ____________________

C. ____________________

14. What is the function of the detrusor muscle?

____

____

____

____

15. What are the functional units of the kidney, and approximately how many are located within each kidney? ____________________

____

____

____

____

Exercise B – Pathology

1. List two possible causes for Cushing's syndrome and the possible treatments for each.

A. ____________________

B. ____________________

2. What is pheochromocytoma? List the classic symptoms. ____________________

____

____

____

3. List the four basic chemical types of urinary calculi and their causes.

A. ____________________

____

B. ____________________

____

C. ____________________

____

D. ____________________

____

4. What is the recurrence rate of urinary calculi? What can be done to reduce the possibility of recurrence?

____

____

____

5. Why is family history an important factor in the diagnosis of PKD? ____________________

____

____

____

____

6. Name two conditions of the kidney that often lead to ESRD.

A. ____________________

B. ____________________

7. What are the two treatment options for a patient with ESRD?

A. ____________________

B. ____________________

8. What age group is most commonly affected by BPH? Why? ____________________

9. Is it possible for hypospadias to occur in a female patient? ____________________

10. List two complications that may occur if cryptorchidism is undiagnosed or untreated.

A. ____________________

B. ____________________

11. What is the normal blood level of PSA? Does an elevated PSA indicate the presence of a malignant process? ____________________

12. An IVU has been unsuccessful in demonstrating a ureteral obstruction. What diagnostic exam may be recommended as the next step? ____________________

13. Table 20-6 in the textbook lists the abnormal constituents of urine. If a patient exhibits an increase in leukocytes, what condition(s) could this indicate?

14. What condition is the MIBG nuclear medicine study designed to detect? ____________________

15. What is KUB? What information may be provided during this type of exam? ____________________

Exercise C – Operation

1. A retrograde urogram is considered a diagnostic radiographic procedure. Why is it often performed in the operating room rather than the radiology department? ____________________

2. List at least three features of the Cysto Room that may not be found in the general OR. ____________________

3. What is the function of a deflecting mechanism?

4. What is the purpose of an O'Connor shield?

5. What specific structure is the Gibson incision designed to access?

6. In which position is the patient placed when use of a flank incision is anticipated?

7. List the three flank incision options and give a brief description of the location of each.

A.

B.

C.

8. What is the purpose of renal cooling?

9. Why is it important for the STSR to have a chest tube, insertion supplies, and a water-seal drainage system readily available during a nephrectomy?

10. List the three sources from which kidneys are obtained for transplant.

A.

B.

C.

11. What is the purpose of suprapubic cystostomy?

12. Will the surgical technologist be scrubbed in for cystoscopy? What is the main function of the surgical technologist during cystoscopy?

13. List four procedures that may be performed transurethrally.

A.

B.

C.

D.

14. Why is it necessary for the assistant to change the gloves (and possibly the gown) during MMK?

____

____

____

____

15. What is the purpose of repeatedly introducing the cystoscope during a Stamey procedure?__________

____

____

____

____

Exercise D – Specific Variations

Student Name ______________________ Date ______________

Instructor ______________________

Surgical Procedure – Student Case Study Report

The student will be provided with basic patient information (real or simulated) and is expected to complete the following case study.

1. Procedure name: ______________________
2. Definition of procedure: ______________________
3. What is the purpose of the procedure? ______________________
4. What is the expected outcome of the procedure?
5. Patient age: ______________________
6. Gender: ______________________
7. Additional pertinent patient information: ______________________
8. Probable preoperative diagnosis: ______________________
9. How was the diagnosis determined? ______________________
10. Discuss the relevant anatomy. ______________________
11. List the general and procedure-specific equipment that will be needed for the procedure.

12. List the general and procedure-specific instruments that will be needed for the procedure.

13. List the basic and procedure-specific supplies that will be needed for the procedure.

Pack

Basin

Gloves

Blades

Drapes

Drains

Dressings

Suture—Type of Suture, Needle (if applicable), and Anticipated Tissue Usage

Pharmaceuticals

Miscellaneous

14. Operative preparation:

15. What type of anesthesia will likely be used? Why?

16. List any special anesthesia equipment that may be needed.

17. Patient position during the procedure:

18. What supplies will be necessary for positioning?

19. What type of shave/skin preparation will be necessary (if any)?

20. Define the anatomic perimeters of the prep.

21. List the order in which the drapes will be applied, and describe any specific variations.

22. List any practical considerations.

23. List the procedural steps, and describe the preparatory and supportive actions of the STSR during each step (use additional space if necessary).

Operative Procedure	Technical Considerations
1.	•
	•
2.	•
	•
3.	•
	•
4.	•
	•
5.	•
	•

(continues)

Operative Procedure *(continued)*	**Technical Considerations** *(continued)*
6.	•
	•
7.	•
	•
8.	•
	•
9.	•
	•
10.	•
	•

24. What is the postoperative diagnosis? ______________

25. Describe the immediate postoperative care.

26. What is the patient's long-term prognosis?

27. What are the possible complications? ______________

28. Comments or questions: ______________

29. What is the most valuable information you obtained from preparing this surgical procedure case study?

Case Studies

☐ CASE STUDY 1

Patricia has been experiencing several seemingly unrelated symptoms that include weight loss, headache, "heartburn," sweating, trembling, rapid heart rate, heat intolerance, and a feeling of anxiousness. Patricia's daughter finally convinced her to see her primary care physician, who has determined that Patricia has a tumor of the adrenal medulla.

1. What diagnostic studies are needed to confirm the diagnosis?

____

____

____

____

2. What is the name of Patricia's tumor, and how serious is it? Why?

____

____

____

____

3. What is the necessary treatment for Patricia's condition? What type of procedure will most likely be performed?

____

____

____

____

☐

☐ CASE STUDY 2

Six-year-old Belinda has been suffering from chronic urinary tract infections. The appearance of blood in her urine led to further testing that produced a diagnosis of PKD. Belinda's condition has nearly destroyed both kidneys. Belinda, her parents, and her twin sister, Melinda, are all extremely concerned about Belinda's future.

1. What does PKD mean, and from what type of PKD does Belinda suffer? ______________________

2. What does the term *parenchyma* mean? What are the parenchymatous organs? ______________________

3. Was invasive testing necessary to determine Belinda's diagnosis? ______________________

4. What course is the disease expected to follow? ______________________

5. What will be the most likely outcome for Belinda? ______________________

☐

CHAPTER 21

Orthopedic Surgery

OBJECTIVES

After studying this chapter, the reader should be able to:

A 1. Discuss the relevant anatomy and physiology of the musculoskeletal system.

P 2. Describe the pathology of the musculoskeletal system that prompts surgical intervention and the related terminology.

3. Discuss any special preoperative orthopedic diagnostic procedures/tests.

O 4. Discuss any special preoperative preparation related to orthopedic procedures.

5. Identify the names and uses of orthopedic instruments, supplies, and drugs.

6. Identify the names and uses of special equipment related to orthopedic procedures.

7. Discuss the intraoperative preparation of the patient undergoing an orthopedic procedure.

8. Define and give an overview of the orthopedic procedure.

9. Discuss the purpose and expected outcomes of the orthopedic procedure.

10. Discuss the immediate postoperative care and possible complications of the orthopedic procedure.

S 11. Discuss any specific variations related to the preoperative, intraoperative, and postoperative care of the orthopedic patient.

Key Terms

Define the following:

1. abduction ______________________________
____
2. AC joint ______________________________
____
3. adduction ______________________________
____
4. amphiarthrosis ______________________________
____
5. cancellous bone ______________________________
____
6. cartilage ______________________________
____
7. comminuted ______________________________
____
8. compound fracture ______________________________
____
9. cortical bone ______________________________
____
10. diarthrosis ______________________________
____
11. epiphysis ______________________________
____
12. flexion ______________________________
____
13. ligament ______________________________
____
14. marrow ______________________________
____
15. osteogenesis ______________________________
____
16. pedicle ______________________________
____
17. proximal ______________________________
____
18. shoulder joint ______________________________
____
19. splint ______________________________
____
20. valgus ______________________________
____

Exercise A – Anatomy

1. Identify the skeletal bones shown in Figure 21-1.

A. ______________________

B. ______________________

C. ______________________

D. ______________________

E. ______________________

F. ______________________

G. ______________________

H. ______________________

I. ______________________

J. ______________________

K. ______________________

L. ______________________

M. ______________________

N. ______________________

O. ______________________

P. ______________________

Q. ______________________

R. ______________________

S. ______________________

T. ______________________

U. ______________________

V. ______________________

W. ______________________

X. ______________________

Y. ______________________

Z. ______________________

AA. ______________________

BB. ______________________

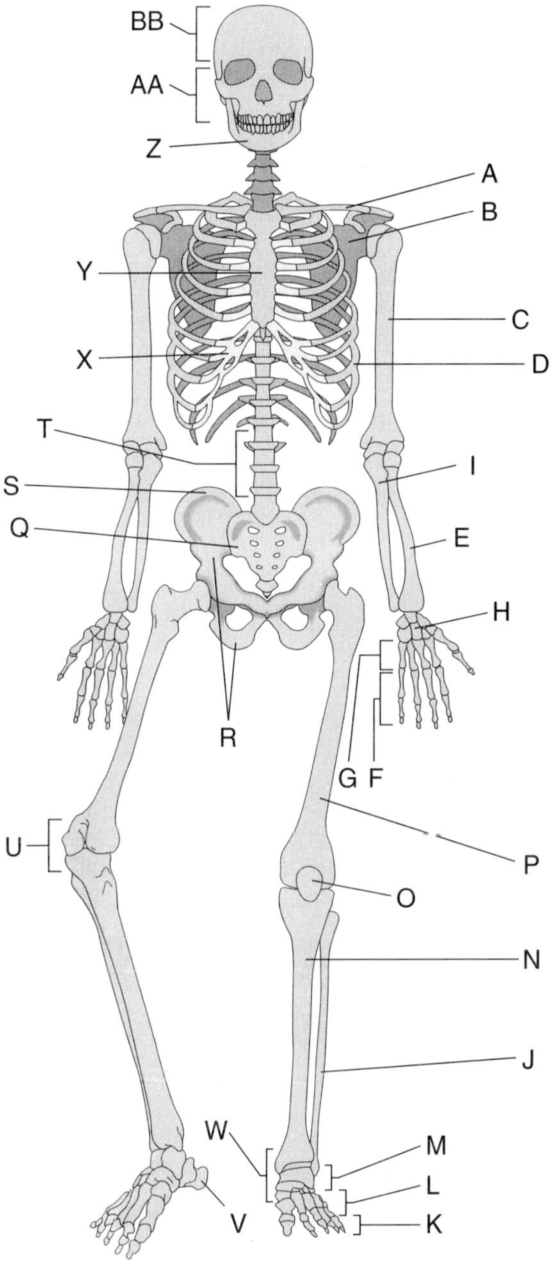

Figure 21-1

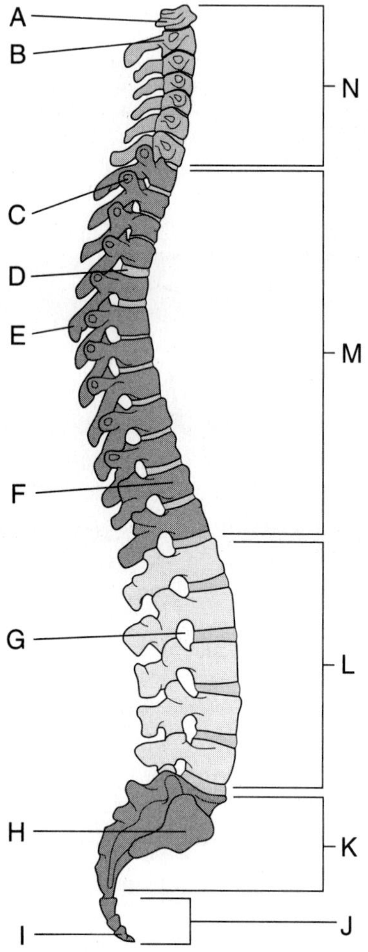

Figure 21-2

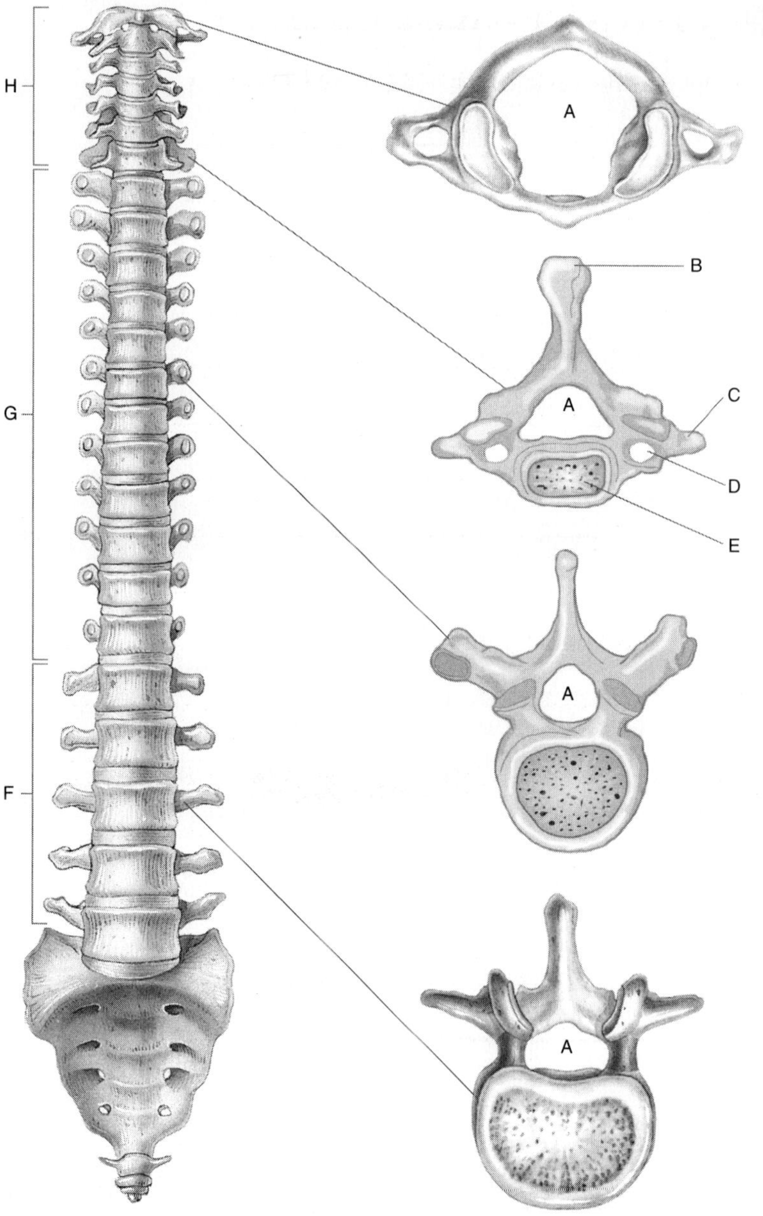

Figure 21-3

2. Identify the structures of the vertebral column shown in Figure 21-2.

A. ____________________

B. ____________________

C. ____________________

D. ____________________

E. ____________________

F. ____________________

G. ____________________

H. ____________________

I. ____________________

J. ____________________

K. ____________________

L. ____________________

M. ____________________

N. ____________________

3. Identify the vertebral structures shown in Figure 21-3.

   A. ______________________

   B. ______________________

   C. ______________________

   D. ______________________

   E. ______________________

   F. ______________________

   G. ______________________

   H. ______________________

4. Identify the structures shown in Figure 21-4.

   A. ______________________

   B. ______________________

   C. ______________________

   D. ______________________

   E. ______________________

   F. ______________________

5. Identify the bones of the pelvic girdle shown in Figure 21-5.

   A. ______________________

   B. ______________________

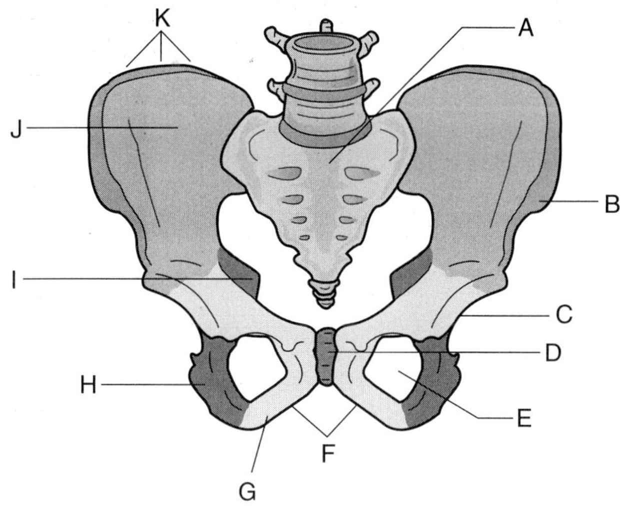

Figure 21-5

   C. ______________________

   D. ______________________

   E. ______________________

   F. ______________________

   G. ______________________

   H. ______________________

   I. ______________________

   J. ______________________

   K. ______________________

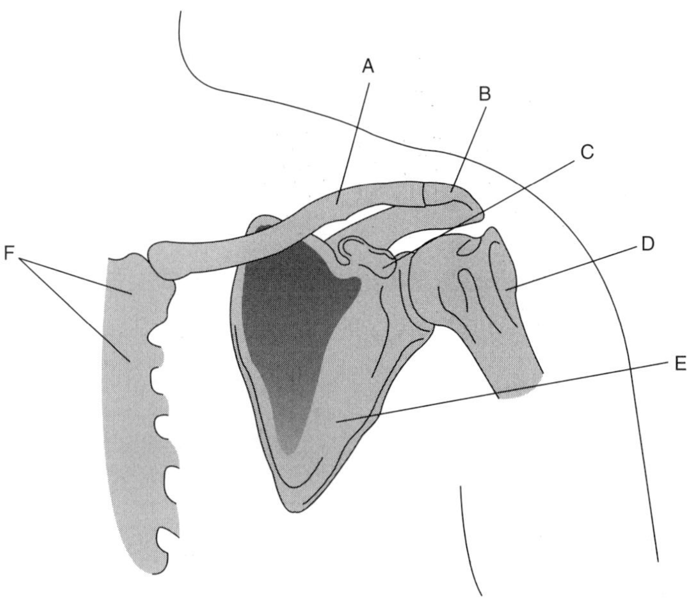

Figure 21-4

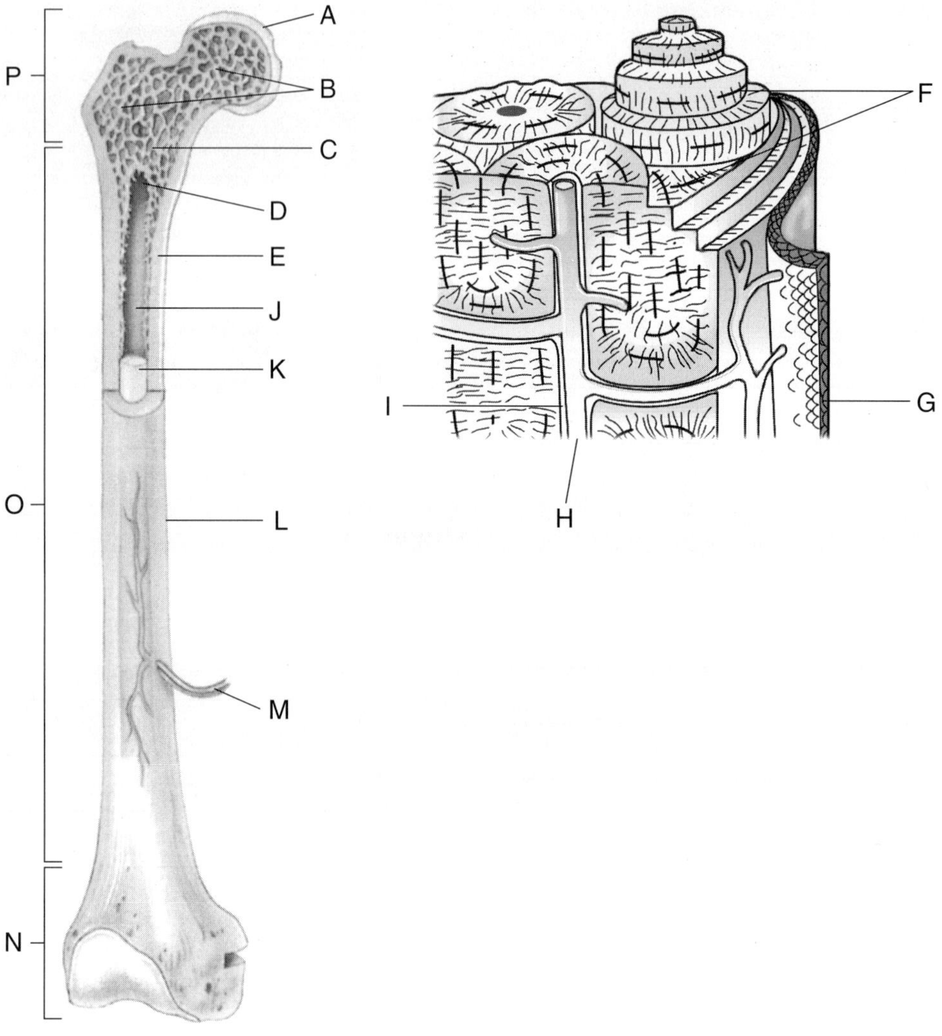

Figure 21-6

6. Identify the elements of a long bone as shown in Figure 21-6.

A. ______________________

B. ______________________

C. ______________________

D. ______________________

E. ______________________

F. ______________________

G. ______________________

H. ______________________

I. ______________________

J. ______________________

K. ______________________

L. ______________________

M. ______________________

N. ______________________

O. ______________________

P. ______________________

7. List the five functions of the skeletal system.

A. ______

B. ______

C. ______

D. ______

E. ______

8. List four factors that affect bone growth.

A. ______

B. ______

C. ______

D. ______

9. Define the term *sesamoid,* and give two examples of sesamoid bones. ______

______

______

A. ______

B. ______

10. What are the two main divisions of the skeleton? Briefly describe each division.

A. ______

______

B. ______

______

11. List the eight bones of the cranium.

A. ______

B. ______

C. ______

D. ______

E. ______

F. ______

G. ______

H. ______

12. Name the three bones that comprise the knee joint.

A. ______

B. ______

C. ______

13. Describe the function of a gliding joint, and provide an example of a gliding joint. ______

______

______

______

______

______

14. Define circumduction, and give an example of a joint that is capable of circumduction. ______

______

______

______

______

______

15. In addition to calcium, name four other minerals that are stored within bone.

A. ______

B. ______

C. ______

D. ______

Exercise B – Pathology

1. What is ankylosis, and what is its cause? ______

______

______

______

______

______

2. How does vitamin D help to prevent osteomalacia?

3. Describe a greenstick fracture.

4. Does a patient suffering from subluxation have a fracture? Explain your answer.

5. Describe nonunion, and provide two reasons why nonunion may occur.

6. What is the cause of compartmental syndrome? How is compartmental syndrome manifested?

7. Why is the Lachman and Drawer examination performed?

8. What is the main complication of osteoporosis?

9. What bone is affected by a Colles' fracture?

10. A tumor of the cartilage is called a(n) ________

11. What is the most common type of meniscal tear? Describe the defect.

12. ________ is an inflammation of the bone and bone marrow.

13. An elevated erythrocyte sedimentation rate (ESR) is an indicator of what type of condition?

14. What muscles comprise the rotator cuff? How will a tear of one or more of these muscles or their tendinous attachments affect the shoulder?

15. An arthrogram is an X-ray of what specific structure(s)? ____________

Exercise C – Operation

1. What is meant by the term *exsanguination*? How does this apply to extremity surgery with the use of a tourniquet? ____________

2. What is the maximum recommended time that tourniquet pressure may be applied to an upper extremity? Why? ____________

3. What are two advantages to postoperative use of the CPM machine?

   A. ____________

   B. ____________

4. What precautions must be taken when the use of a C-Arm is expected? ____________

5. Describe the direction of the blade motion of a reciprocating saw. ____________

6. What is bone wax, and how is it used? ____________

7. List two situations in which a bone graft may be required.

   A. ____________

   B. ____________

8. What is the reason for application of irrigation fluid to the wound when sawing or drilling bone?

9. When using MMA, what is the importance of using a closed mixing system? ____________

10. What information must be documented following prosthesis insertion?

    A. ____________

    B. ____________

    C. ____________

    D. ____________

11. List two reasons why arthroscopy may be performed.

A. ______________________________

B. ______________________________

12. What is a reamer used to accomplish?

____

____

____

____

13. What are the three main advantages of maintaining laminar airflow in the OR during a surgical procedure?

A. ______________________________

B. ______________________________

C. ______________________________

14. Following closed reduction, what method of immobilization is commonly employed? ______________

____

____

____

____

____

15. List the three types of traction.

A. ______________________________

B. ______________________________

C. ______________________________

Exercise D – Specific Variations

Student Name ______________________ Date ______________

Instructor ______________________

Surgical Procedure – Student Case Study Report

The student will be provided with basic patient information (real or simulated) and is expected to complete the following case study.

1. Procedure name: ______________________

2. Definition of procedure: ______________________

3. What is the purpose of the procedure? ______________________

4. What is the expected outcome of the procedure?

5. Patient age: ______________________

6. Gender: ______________________

7. Additional pertinent patient information: ______________________

8. Probable preoperative diagnosis: ______________________

9. How was the diagnosis determined? ______________________

10. Discuss the relevant anatomy. ______________________

11. List the general and procedure-specific equipment that will be needed for the procedure.

12. List the general and procedure-specific instruments that will be needed for the procedure.

13. List the basic and procedure-specific supplies that will be needed for the procedure.

Pack

Basin

Gloves

Blades

Drapes

Drains

Dressings

Suture—Type of Suture, Needle (if applicable), and Anticipated Tissue Usage

Pharmaceuticals

Miscellaneous

14. Operative preparation:

15. What type of anesthesia will likely be used? Why?

16. List any special anesthesia equipment that may be needed.

17. Patient position during the procedure:

18. What supplies will be necessary for positioning?

____

____

____

____

____

19. What type of shave/skin preparation will be necessary (if any)? ___________________________

____

____

____

____

____

20. Define the anatomic perimeters of the prep.

____

____

____

____

____

21. List the order in which the drapes will be applied, and describe any specific variations.

____

____

____

____

____

22. List any practical considerations.

____

____

____

____

____

____

23. List the procedural steps, and describe the preparatory and supportive actions of the STSR during each step (use additional space if necessary).

Operative Procedure	Technical Considerations
1.	•
	•
2.	•
	•
3.	•
	•
4.	•
	•
5.	•
	•

(continues)

Operative Procedure *(continued)*	Technical Considerations *(continued)*
6.	•
	•
7.	•
	•
8.	•
	•
9.	•
	•
10.	•
	•

24. What is the postoperative diagnosis? ______________

25. Describe the immediate postoperative care.

26. What is the patient's long-term prognosis?

27. What are the possible complications? ______________

28. Comments or questions: ______________

29. What is the most valuable information you obtained from preparing this surgical procedure case study?

Case Studies

☐ CASE STUDY 1

Ellenor is a 65-year-old female who was admitted to the hospital for a total hip arthroplasty.

1. Describe a routine draping procedure for this case. ______________________________

2. What kind of incision is used? ______________________________

3. After the femoral osteotomy guide is placed over the lateral femur and neck, what should the STSR plan to do next? ______________________________

4. Will the incision be drained? ______________________________

5. Describe the immediate postoperative care the patient will receive. ______________________________

☐

☐ CASE STUDY 2

Leroy was admitted to the emergency department with a fracture of the left tibia and fibula. The fracture was reduced, the leg placed in a cast, and Leroy was sent home.

1. Why are casts placed on limbs with reduced fractures? ______________________________

2. What is the meaning of the term ***distraction***? What complications can be caused by distraction? ______________________________

3. What is the most important factor in bone healing? ______________________________

4. To what does the term ***delayed union*** refer? ______________________________

☐

CHAPTER 22

Cardiothoracic Surgery

OBJECTIVES

After studying this chapter, the reader should be able to:

A 1. Discuss the relevant anatomy of the cardiovascular and respiratory systems.

P 2. Describe the pathology that prompts cardiac or thoracic surgical intervention and the related terminology.

3. Discuss any special preoperative diagnostic procedures/tests for the patient undergoing cardiac or thoracic surgery.

O 4. Discuss any special preoperative preparation procedures.

5. Identify the names and uses of cardiovascular and thoracic instruments, supplies, and drugs.

6. Identify the names and uses of special equipment for the cardiac or thoracic procedure.

7. Discuss the intraoperative preparation of the patient undergoing a cardiac or thoracic procedure.

8. Define and give an overview of the cardiac or thoracic procedure.

9. Discuss the purpose and expected outcomes of the cardiac or thoracic procedure.

10. Discuss the immediate postoperative care and possible complications of the cardiac or thoracic procedure.

S 11. Discuss any specific variations related to the preoperative, intraoperative, and postoperative care of the patient undergoing a cardiac or thoracic procedure.

Select Key Terms

Define the following:

1. alveoli ______________________________
2. aneurysm ______________________________
3. arrhythmia ______________________________
4. atria ______________________________
5. bradycardia ______________________________
6. cardiac cycle ______________________________
7. ductus arteriosus ______________________________
8. hyaline cartilage ______________________________
9. infarction ______________________________
10. infiltrate ______________________________
11. mediastinum ______________________________
12. myocardium ______________________________
13. oxygenated ______________________________
14. pericardium ______________________________
15. pleura ______________________________
16. prolapse ______________________________
17. PVC ______________________________
18. regurgitation ______________________________
19. stent ______________________________
20. systole ______________________________
21. tachycardia ______________________________
22. tamponade ______________________________
23. ventricles ______________________________

Exercise A – Anatomy

1. Identify the structures shown in Figure 22-1.

A. ______________________________

B. ______________________________

C. ______________________________

D. ______________________________

E. ______________________________

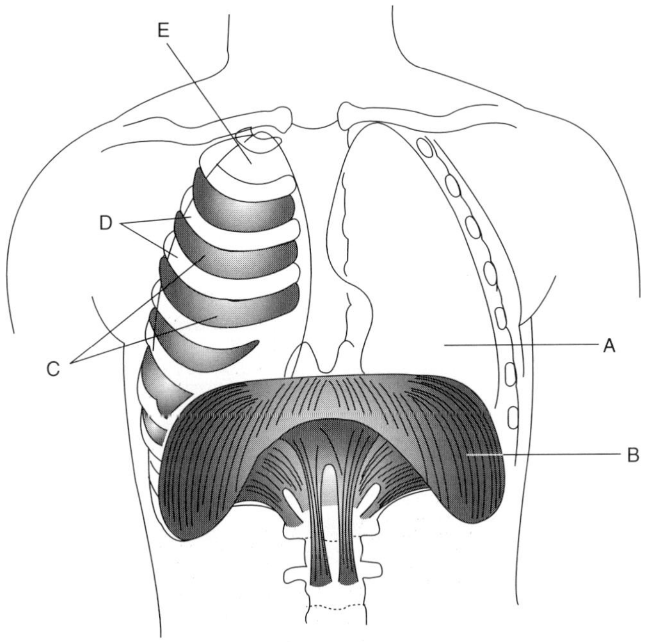

Figure 22-1

2. Identify the structures shown in Figure 22-2.

A. ______________________________

B. ______________________________

C. ______________________________

D. ______________________________

E. ______________________________

F. ______________________________

G. ______________________________

H. ______________________________

I. ______________________________

J. ______________________________

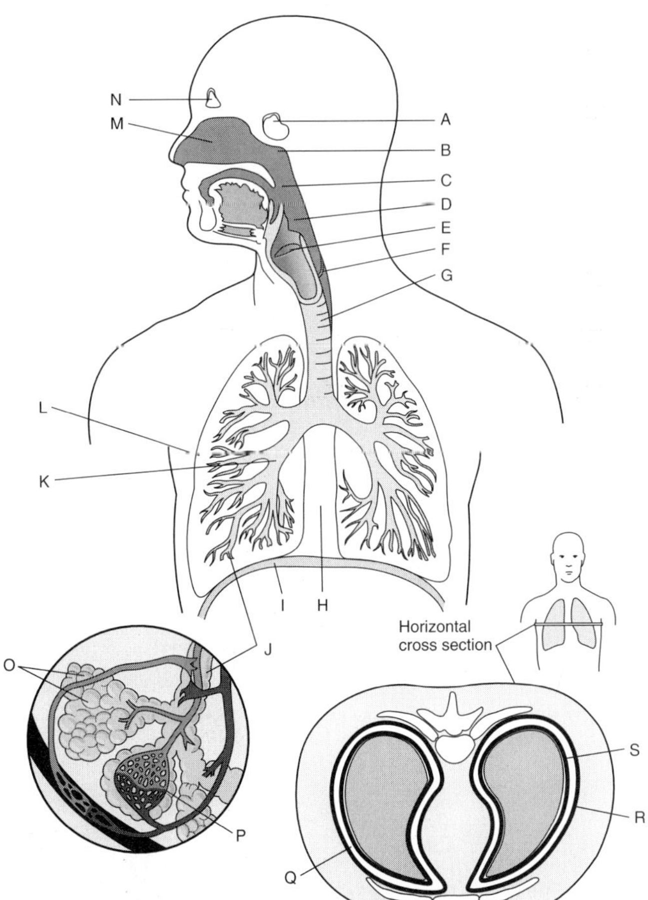

Figure 22-2

K. ____________________

L. ____________________

M. ____________________

N. ____________________

O. ____________________

P. ____________________

Q. ____________________

R. ____________________

S. ____________________

3. Identify the structures shown in Figure 22-3.

A. ____________________

B. ____________________

C. ____________________

D. ____________________

E. ____________________

F. ____________________

G. ____________________

H. ____________________

I. ____________________

J. ____________________

K. ____________________

L. ____________________

M. ____________________

N. ____________________

O. ____________________

P. ____________________

Q. ____________________

R. ____________________

S. ____________________

T. ____________________

U. ____________________

V. ____________________

W. ____________________

X. ____________________

Y. ____________________

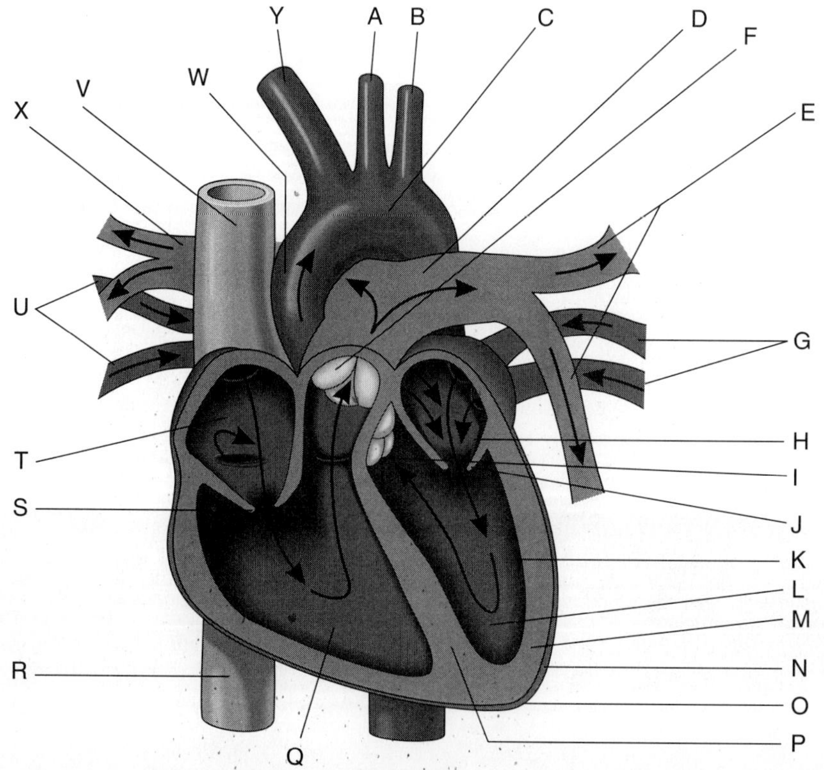

Figure 22-3

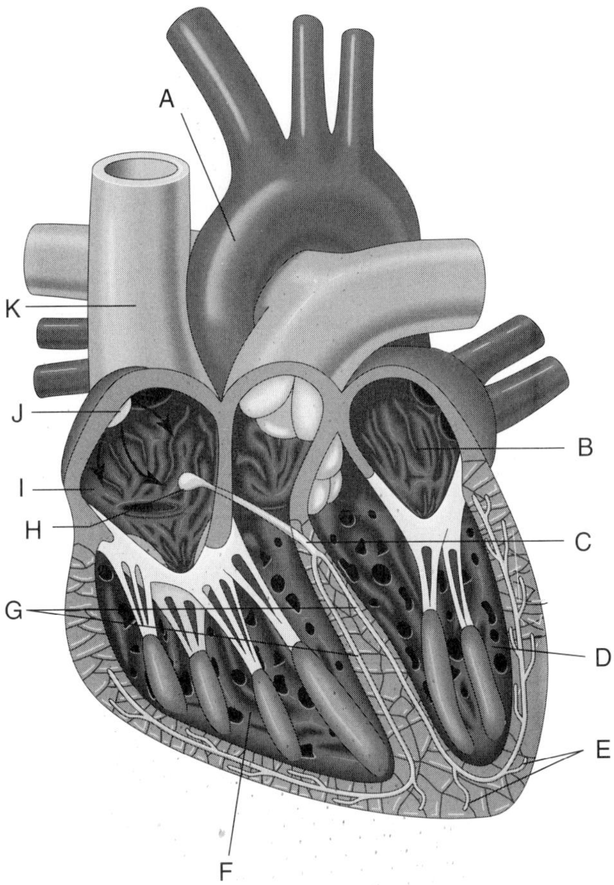

Figure 22-4

4. Identify the structures shown in Figure 22-4.

A. ____________________

B. ____________________

C. ____________________

D. ____________________

E. ____________________

F. ____________________

G. ____________________

H. ____________________

I. ____________________

J. ____________________

K. ____________________

5. Identify the cardiac valves shown in Figure 22-5.

A. ____________________

B. ____________________

C. ____________________

6. Identify the structures shown in Figure 22-6.

A. ____________________

B. ____________________

C. ____________________

D. ____________________

E. ____________________

F. ____________________

G. ____________________

H. ____________________

I. ____________________

J. ____________________

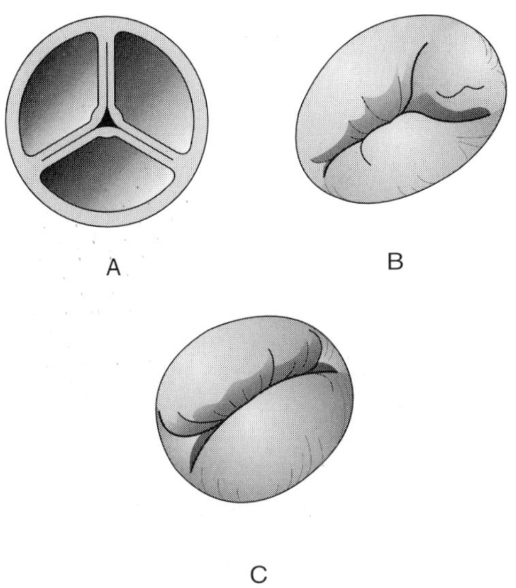

Figure 22-5

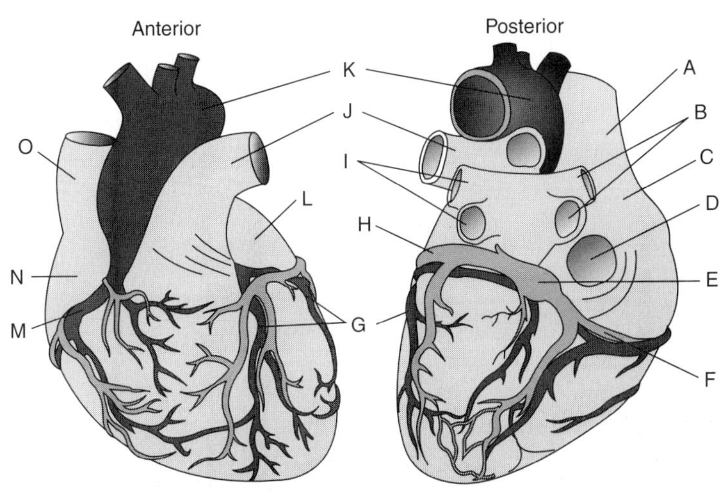

Figure 22-6

K. ______________________________

L. ______________________________

M. ______________________________

N. ______________________________

O. ______________________________

7. List the following events in the proper chronological sequence to complete the cardiac cycle.

A. ______________ Atria contract

B. ______________ AV node stimulated

C. ______________ Impulse moves through right and left bundle branches

D. ______________ Impulse transmitted to bundle of His

E. ______________ Impulse travels via internodal atrial pathways

F. ______________ Purkinje fibers stimulated

G. ______________ SA node generates initial impulse

H. ______________ Ventricles contract

8. Trace the flow of blood from the time it leaves the venae cavae to the time it enters the aorta by placing the following elements in the correct order.

A. ______________ Aorta

B. ______________ Aortic (semilunar) valve

C. ______________ Bicuspid (mitral) valve

D. ______________ Left atrium

E. ______________ Left ventricle

F. ______________ Lungs

G. ______________ Pulmonary arteries

H. ______________ Pulmonary valve

I. ______________ Pulmonary veins

J. ______________ Right atrium

K. ______________ Right ventricle

L. ______________ Tricuspid (right AV) valve

M. ______________ Venae cavae

9. Name the three layers of the heart wall.

A. ______________________________

B. ______________________________

C. ______________________________

10. Name the four cardiac valves and describe their locations.

A. ______________________________

____

B. ______________________________

____

C. ______________________________

____

D. ______________________________

____

11. Define cardiac output. ______________

____

____

____

12. What is the function of the bundle of His?

____

____

____

____

13. Name and describe the two layers of the pleura.

A. ______________________________

____

B. ______________________________

____

14. What structures are contained within the mediastinum? ______________

____

____

____

____

15. Name the principal muscles of inspiration.

A. ______

B. ______

Exercise B – Pathology

1. List three methods used to detect lung tumors.

A. ______

B. ______

C. ______

2. Describe the condition known as flail chest.

______

3. Penetrating chest trauma will result in which condition? What treatment is necessary? ______

4. What is cardiac tamponade? What treatment is necessary? ______

5. List the three types of thoracic outlet syndrome and the cause of each.

A. ______

B. ______

C. ______

6. Describe a Type II dissecting aneurysm of the thoracic aorta. What does dissecting mean in reference to an aneurysm? ______

7. What is the composition of an atheroma? What causes formation of an atheroma? ______

8. Which cardiac enzyme levels rise following myocardial infarction?

A. ______

B. ______

C. ______

9. List three complications of myocardial infarction.

A. ______

B. ______

C. ______

10. What effect does alcohol have on cardiac tissue?

______

11. Describe the condition known as patent ductus arteriosus, list the symptoms, and provide treatment options. ______

12. List the four cardiac defects seen in the classic form of tetralogy of Fallot.

A. ______

B. ______

C. ______

D. ______

13. List two variable and two inherited risk factors for coronary atherosclerosis.

A. ______

B. ______

C. ______

D. ______

14. What is/are the cause(s) of mitral regurgitation?

______

15. A commissurotomy is performed to treat which condition? ______

Exercise C – Operation

1. List the two types of mediastinoscopy, and provide a brief description of each.

A. ______

B. ______

2. Is bronchoscopy strictly a diagnostic procedure? Explain your answer. ______

3. In which position will the patient be placed in order to accomplish a posterolateral thoracotomy?

______

4. Explain the difference between lobectomy and pneumonectomy. ______

5. What is the purpose of inserting a double-lumen endotracheal tube during a thoracotomy?

______

6. In which position will the patient be placed to accomplish a median sternotomy? ______

7. What is empyema? What procedure is performed to treat empyema? ______

8. Which body functions are taken over by the pump oxygenator during open-heart surgery?

______

9. Describe the placement of the cannulas necessary for a cardiopulmonary bypass. ______________________

____

____

____

____

10. Name two blood vessels that are most commonly used as the graft during CABG procedures.

A. ____

B. ____

11. List the two basic types of materials that are used for cardiac valve replacement.

A. ____

B. ____

12. What are the two main components of a pacemaker?

A. ____

B. ____

13. Why is it important to have an open-heart team on "standby" during PTCA? ______________________

____

____

____

____

14. Is cardiopulmonary bypass necessary for closure of a patent ductus arteriosus in an infant?

____

____

____

____

15. What is the purpose of administering potassium cardioplegia solution during open-heart procedures? __

____

____

____

____

Exercise D – Specific Variations

Student Name ______________________ Date ____________

Instructor ______________________

Surgical Procedure – Student Case Study Report

The student will be provided with basic patient information (real or simulated) and is expected to complete the following case study.

1. Procedure name: ______________________
2. Definition of procedure: ______________________
3. What is the purpose of the procedure? ______________________
4. What is the expected outcome of the procedure?
5. Patient age: ______________________
6. Gender: ______________________
7. Additional pertinent patient information: ______________________
8. Probable preoperative diagnosis: ______________________
9. How was the diagnosis determined? ______________________
10. Discuss the relevant anatomy. ______________________
11. List the general and procedure-specific equipment that will be needed for the procedure.

12. List the general and procedure-specific instruments that will be needed for the procedure.

13. List the basic and procedure-specific supplies that will be needed for the procedure.

Pack

Basin

Gloves

Blades

Drapes

Drains

Dressings

Suture—Type of Suture, Needle (if applicable), and Anticipated Tissue Usage

Pharmaceuticals

Miscellaneous

14. Operative preparation:

15. What type of anesthesia will likely be used? Why?

16. List any special anesthesia equipment that may be needed.

17. Patient position during the procedure:

18. What supplies will be necessary for positioning?

____

____

____

____

____

19. What type of shave/skin preparation will be necessary (if any)?______________________________

____

____

____

____

____

20. Define the anatomic perimeters of the prep.

____

____

____

____

____

21. List the order in which the drapes will be applied, and describe any specific variations.

____

____

____

____

____

22. List any practical considerations.

____

____

____

____

____

____

23. List the procedural steps, and describe the preparatory and supportive actions of the STSR during each step (use additional space if necessary).

Operative Procedure	Technical Considerations
1.	•
	•
2.	•
	•
3.	•
	•
4.	•
	•
5.	•
	•
6.	•
	•

Operative Procedure *(continued)*	Technical Considerations *(continued)*
7.	•
	•
8.	•
	•
9.	•
	•
10.	•
	•

24. What is the postoperative diagnosis? ____________

25. Describe the immediate postoperative care.

26. What is the patient's long-term prognosis?

27. What are the possible complications? ____________

28. Comments or questions: ____________

29. What is the most valuable information you obtained from preparing this surgical procedure case study?

Case Studies

CASE STUDY 1

Elroy has been transported to the emergency department following a motor vehicle accident (MVA). He was the unrestrained driver of one of the vehicles, and his body hit the steering wheel on impact. Elroy has dyspnea, tachypnea, and tachycardia, appears extremely anxious, and is showing signs of shock. Upon examination, the emergency physician notes distant heart sounds, hypotension, and jugular venous distension. A Swan-Ganz catheter placed by the physician reveals equal RA and pulmonary capillary wedge pressures and an elevated CVP.

1. What type of injury is suspected as a result of the blunt chest trauma? ______________________________

2. What diagnostic exams are indicated? ______________________________

3. What is the treatment for this condition? ______________________________

☐ CASE STUDY 2

Timothy, a 49-year-old construction worker, fell from a scaffold and was rushed to the emergency department, where he was evaluated by the trauma team. Timothy complained of chest pain, and severe respiratory distress was noted by the physician. Chest X-ray revealed fractures of the fifth and sixth ribs on the right and absence of lung markings over the affected area.

1. In addition to Timothy's fractured ribs, what other condition is affecting him? ______________________

2. What treatment will be provided? ______________________

3. What type of wound drainage system will be needed? Why? ______________________

4. Will a wound dressing be necessary? If so, what type and why? ______________________

CHAPTER 23

Peripheral Vascular Surgery

OBJECTIVES

After studying this chapter, the reader should be able to:

A 1. Discuss the relevant anatomy of the peripheral vascular system.

P 2. Describe the pathology that prompts surgical intervention of the peripheral vascular system and the related terminology.

3. Discuss any special preoperative peripheral vascular diagnostic procedures.

O 4. Discuss any special preoperative preparation procedures.

5. Identify the names and uses of peripheral vascular instruments, supplies, and drugs.

6. Identify the names and uses of special equipment.

7. Discuss the intraoperative preparation of the patient undergoing the peripheral vascular procedure.

8. Define and give an overview of the peripheral vascular procedure.

9. Discuss the purpose and expected outcomes of the peripheral vascular procedure.

10. Discuss the immediate postoperative care and possible complications of the peripheral vascular procedure.

S 11. Discuss any specific variations related to the preoperative, intraoperative, and postoperative care of the patient undergoing peripheral vascular surgery.

Select Key Terms

Define the following:

1. adventitia ______
2. bifurcation ______
3. capillary ______
4. claudication ______
5. contralateral ______
6. diastole ______
7. embolus ______
8. Fogarty catheter ______
9. in situ ______
10. innominate ______
11. intima ______
12. ischemia ______
13. mitigate ______
14. morbidity ______
15. mortality ______
16. occlusion ______
17. papaverine ______
18. patency ______
19. phrenic ______
20. pledget ______
21. plethysmography ______
22. sinus ______
23. thrombus ______
24. valve ______

Exercise A – Anatomy

1. Identify the branches of the aorta shown in Figure 23-1.

   A. ______
   B. ______
   C. ______
   D. ______
   E. ______
   F. ______
   G. ______
   H. ______
   I. ______
   J. ______

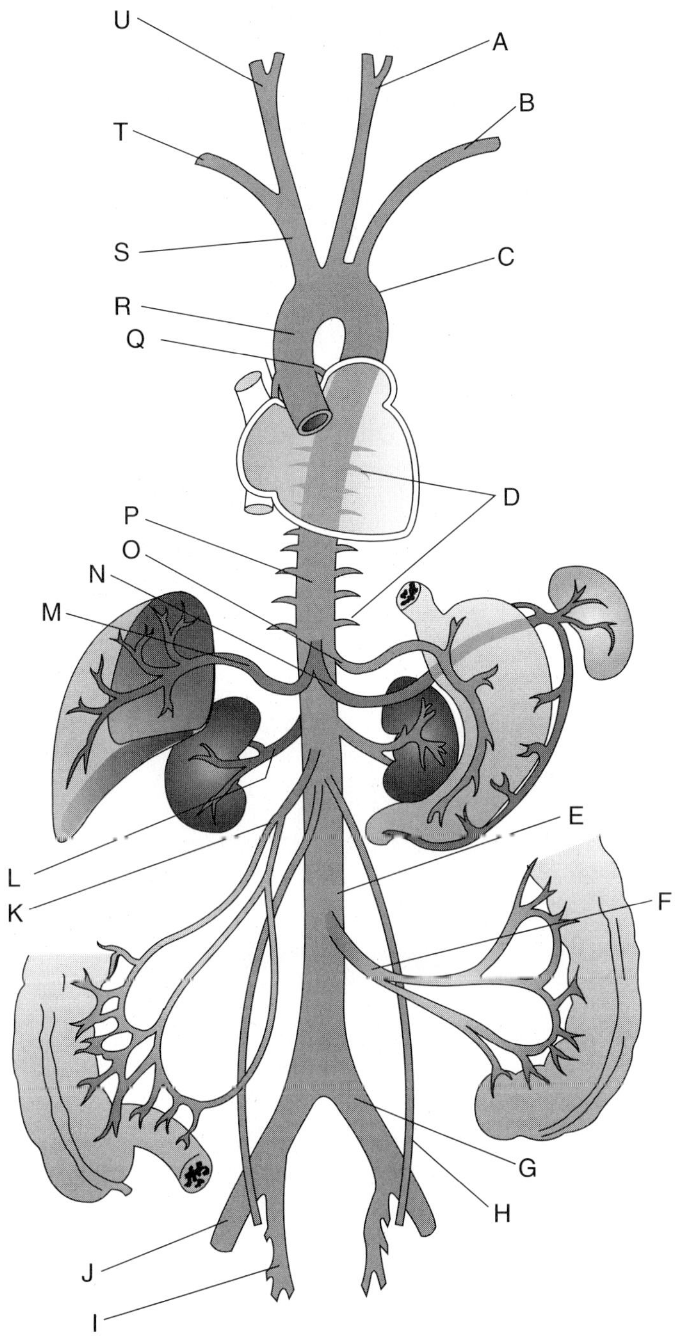

Figure 23-1

K. ______________________

L. ______________________

M. ______________________

N. ______________________

O. ______________________

P. ______________________

Q. ______________________

R. ______________________

S. ______________________

T. ______________________

U. ______________________

2. Identify the systemic arteries shown in Figure 23-2.

A. ______________________

B. ______________________

C. ______________________

D. ______________________

E. ______________________

F. ______________________

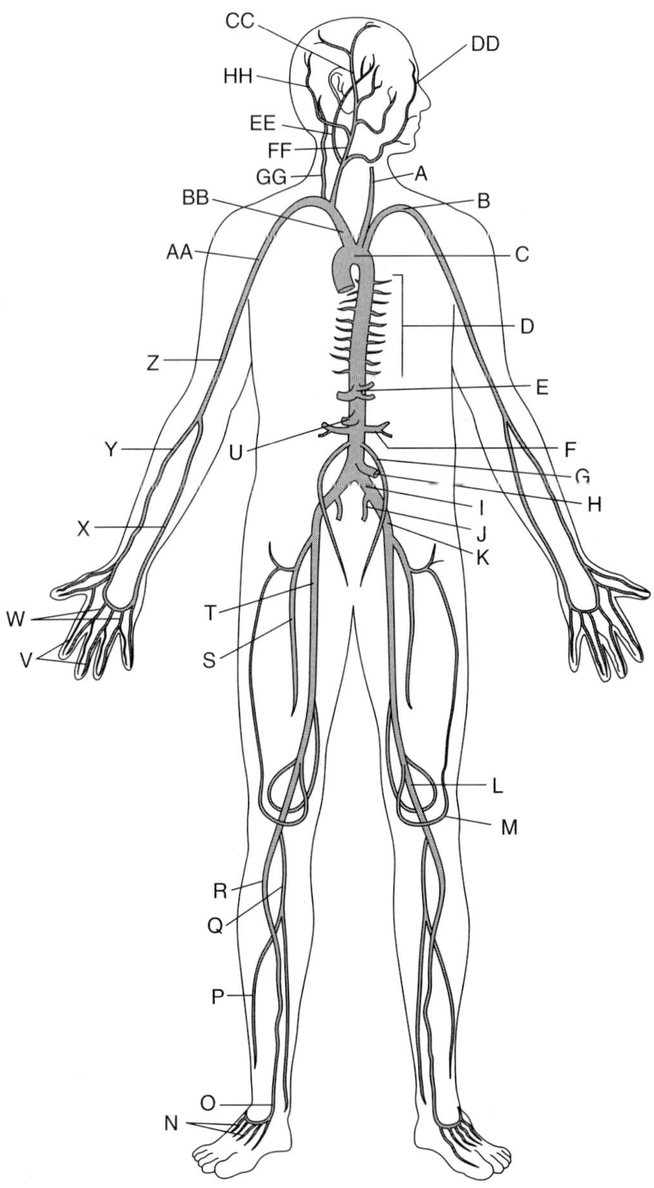

Figure 23-2

G. ______

H. ______

I. ______

J. ______

K. ______

L. ______

M. ______

N. ______

O. ______

P. ______

Q. ______

R. ______

S. ______

T. ______

U. ______

V. ______

W. ______

X. ______

Y. ______

Z. ______

AA. ______

BB. ______

CC. ______

DD. ______

EE. ______

FF. ______

GG. ______

HH. ______

3. Identify the systemic veins shown in Figure 23-3.

A. ______

B. ______

C. ______

D. ______

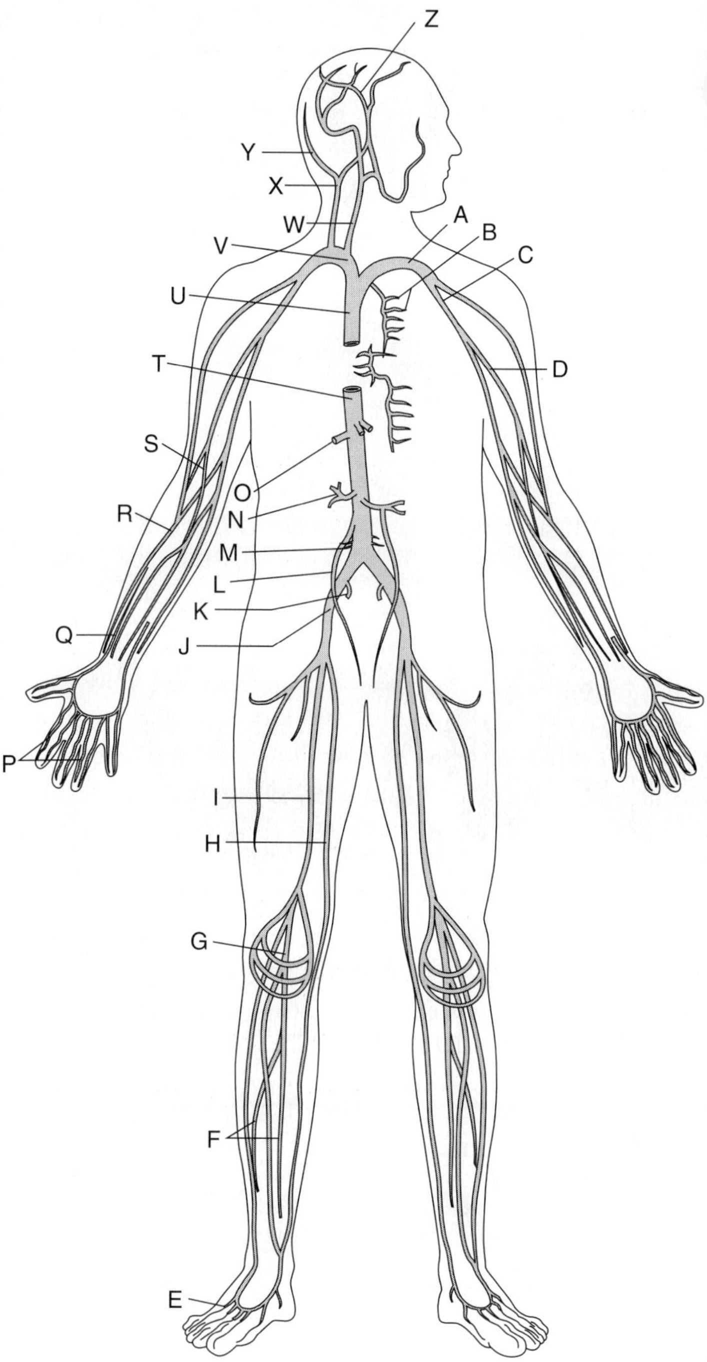

Figure 23-3

E. ______

F. ______

G. ______

H. ______

I. ______

J. ______

K. ______

L. ______________________________

M. ______________________________

N. ______________________________

O. ______________________________

P. ______________________________

Q. ______________________________

R. ______________________________

S. ______________________________

T. ______________________________

U. ______________________________

V. ______________________________

W. ______________________________

X. ______________________________

Y. ______________________________

Z. ______________________________

4. Identify the structures of the blood vessels shown in Figure 23-4.

A. ______________________________

B. ______________________________

C. ______________________________

D. ______________________________

E. ______________________________

F. ______________________________

G. ______________________________

H. ______________________________

I. ______________________________

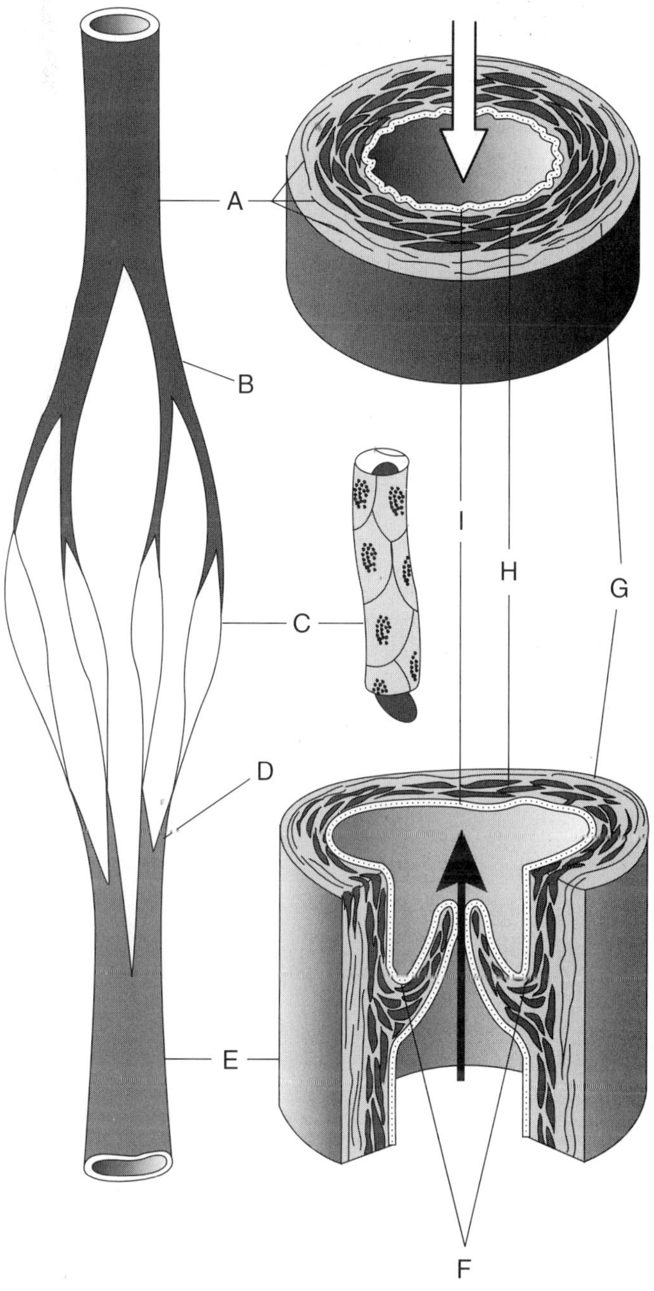

Figure 23-4

5. List the three tunics of a blood vessel wall, and briefly describe the composition and function of each structure.

A. ______________________________

____

B. ______________________________

____

C. ______________________________

____

6. What structures receive arterial blood from the brachiocephalic artery? ______________________________

____

____

____

____

7. Which artery or arteries, if any, branch off the ascending aorta? ______________________________

8. Each common carotid artery bifurcates into two sections. Provide the names of the two branches and the structures supplied with arterial blood from each.

   A. ______________________________

   B. ______________________________

9. What effect does the autonomic nervous system have on vasoconstriction? ______________________________

10. Which is larger, the lumen of an artery or the lumen of a vein in a similar location? ______________________________

11. What effect does vasodilation have on the blood pressure? ______________________________

12. What is blood pressure? ______________________________

13. List three factors that affect arterial blood pressure.

   A. ______________________________

   B. ______________________________

   C. ______________________________

14. What does the term *resistance* describe within the cardiovascular system? How does increased resistance affect blood pressure? ______________________________

15. List the three main branches of the common hepatic artery, and name the structure(s) served by each.

   A. ______________________________

   B. ______________________________

   C. ______________________________

Exercise B – Pathology

1. What causes claudication? ______________________________

2. List the four signs/symptoms of acute arterial occlusion.

   A. ______________________________

   B. ______________________________

   C. ______________________________

   D. ______________________________

3. There are several types of emboli. Name two.

   A. ______________________________

   B. ______________________________

4. List three types of treatment for embolism.

   A. ______________________________

   B. ______________________________

   C. ______________________________

5. What is the shape of a fusiform aneurysm? What portion of the aorta is most often involved?

6. Varicose veins commonly involve the saphenous vein. Describe the condition, and list two possible treatments. ______________________________

7. What term is used to describe inflammation of a vein?

8. What is the cause of a TIA (transient ischemic attack)?

9. What is plaque? ______________________________

10. What examinations may be performed to identify a lesion of the common carotid artery?

11. What is the difference between ischemia and necrosis? ______________________________

12. What are the signs/symptoms associated with a TIA?

13. List four risk factors associated with the development of peripheral vascular disease.

    A. ______________________________

    B. ______________________________

    C. ______________________________

    D. ______________________________

14. How is the establishment of collateral blood flow encouraged in patients with vascular insufficiency of the lower extremity? ______________________________

15. List three physical signs of vascular insufficiency of the lower extremity.

A. ______

B. ______

C. ______

Exercise C – Operation

1. In what situation will contrast solution (e.g., Conray, Hypaque) be needed on the sterile field?

______

2. List three hemostatic agents that are typically used during peripheral vascular surgical procedures.

A. ______

B. ______

C. ______

3. What is a Fogarty catheter used to accomplish?

______

4. What is the purpose of an intraluminal stent?

______

5. Vascular grafts are available in several configurations. Name two.

A. ______

B. ______

6. Why do some types of vascular graft material have rigid rings (exoskeleton) built into the graft? In which location are the reinforced grafts commonly implanted? ______

7. What is the primary indication for carotid endarterectomy? ______

8. During carotid endarterectomy, is the use of a shunt necessary? Why? ______

9. Vascular grafts are available in several materials. Name two.

A. ______

B. ______

10. What instruments are typically used to perform an arteriotomy? ______

11. What is the purpose of creating a tunnel during a femoral popliteal bypass? ______

12. List two complications that may arise following implantation of a composite graft.

A. ______________________

B. ______________________

13. Why is it necessary to pre-clot a vascular graft that is made of knitted polyester? ______________________

____

____

____

____

14. What is a patch suture? How is it prepared?

____

____

____

____

15. Why is it important for the STSR to remain sterile and keep the back table and Mayo stand intact until the patient has been transported to the PACU? ______________________

____

____

____

____

____

____

Exercise D – Specific Variations

Student Name ______________________ Date ______________

Instructor ______________________

Surgical Procedure – Student Case Study Report

The student will be provided with basic patient information (real or simulated) and is expected to complete the following case study.

1. Procedure name: ______________________

2. Definition of procedure: ______________________

3. What is the purpose of the procedure? ______________________

4. What is the expected outcome of the procedure?

5. Patient age: ______________________

6. Gender: ______________________

7. Additional pertinent patient information: ______________________

8. Probable preoperative diagnosis: ______________________

9. How was the diagnosis determined? ______________________

10. Discuss the relevant anatomy. ______________________

11. List the general and procedure-specific equipment that will be needed for the procedure.

12. List the general and procedure-specific instruments that will be needed for the procedure.

13. List the basic and procedure-specific supplies that will be needed for the procedure.

Pack

Basin

Gloves

Blades

Drapes

Drains

Dressings

Suture—Type of Suture, Needle (if applicable), and Anticipated Tissue Usage

Pharmaceuticals

Miscellaneous

14. Operative preparation:

15. What type of anesthesia will likely be used? Why?

16. List any special anesthesia equipment that may be needed.

17. Patient position during the procedure:

18. What supplies will be necessary for positioning?

____

____

____

____

____

19. What type of shave/skin preparation will be necessary (if any)? ______________________

____

____

____

____

____

20. Define the anatomic perimeters of the prep.

____

____

____

____

____

21. List the order in which the drapes will be applied, and describe any specific variations. ______________

____

____

____

____

____

____

22. List any practical considerations. ______________

____

____

____

____

____

23. List the procedural steps, and describe the preparatory and supportive actions of the STSR during each step (use additional space if necessary).

Operative Procedure	Technical Considerations
1.	•
	•
2.	•
	•
3.	•
	•
4.	•
	•
5.	•
	•
6.	•
	•

Operative Procedure *(continued)*	Technical Considerations *(continued)*
7.	•
	•
8.	•
	•
9.	•
	•
10.	•
	•

24. What is the postoperative diagnosis? ____________

25. Describe the immediate postoperative care.

26. What is the patient's long-term prognosis?

27. What are the possible complications? ____________

28. Comments or questions: ____________

29. What is the most valuable information you obtained from preparing this surgical procedure case study?

Case Studies

☐ CASE STUDY 1

Joe is a 50-year-old male who was brought to the emergency department in hemorrhagic shock due to a ruptured abdominal aneurysm. The surgeon called the surgery department to alert them that he is in transit with the patient for immediate intervention. The OR team leader, in turn, has notified the STSR and circulator who are assigned to the case. The surgical team springs into action.

1. What supplies will the STSR open onto the sterile field first? ______________________

2. What instrument sets will be needed? ______________________

3. What instruments will be needed first? ______________________

☐

☐ CASE STUDY 2

Wayne, a 67-year-old male, presented to the emergency department with the following symptoms: severe hypertension, malaise, orthopnea, peripheral edema, and decreased urinary output. He is a pack-a-day smoker and is grossly overweight.

1. What is the preliminary diagnosis? ______________________

2. What diagnostic examination is considered the gold standard for confirmation of the preliminary diagnosis?

3. Will surgical intervention be necessary? If so, what procedure will be scheduled? ______________________

☐

CHAPTER 24 Neurosurgery

OBJECTIVES

After studying this chapter, the reader should be able to:

A 1. Discuss the relevant anatomy and physiology of the neurological system.

P 2. Describe the pathology that prompts surgical intervention of the neurological system and the related terminology.

3. Discuss any special preoperative neurological diagnostic procedures/tests.

O 4. Discuss any special preoperative preparation procedures related to neurosurgery.

5. Identify the names and uses of neurosurgical instruments, supplies, and drugs.

6. Identify the names and uses of special equipment related to neurosurgery.

7. Discuss the intraoperative preparation of the patient undergoing the neurosurgical procedure.

8. Define and give an overview of the neurosurgical procedure.

9. Discuss the purpose and expected outcomes of the neurosurgical procedure.

10. Discuss the immediate postoperative care and possible complications of the neurosurgical procedure.

S 11. Discuss any specific variations related to the preoperative, intraoperative, and postoperative care of the neurosurgical patient.

12. Discuss recent advances in neurosurgery.

Select Key Terms

Define the following:

1. abscess ______________________________

____

2. acute ______________________________

____

3. autonomic nervous system ______________________________

____

4. cerebellum ______________________________

____

5. cerebrum ______________________________

____

6. circle of Willis ______________________________

____

7. CNS ______________________________

____

8. decompress ______________________________

____

9. dysraphism ______________________________

____

10. epidural ______________________________

____

11. extruded ______________________________

____

12. glioma ______________________________

____

13. hematoma ______________________________

____

14. ICP ______________________________

____

15. integration ______________________________

____

16. meninges ______________________________

____

17. osteophyte ______________________________

____

18. parasympathetic nervous system ______________________________

____

19. PNS ______________________________

____

20. radiculopathy ______________________________

____

21. somatic nervous system ______________________________

____

22. sympathetic nervous system ______________________________

____

23. TIA ______________________________

____

24. transphenoidal ______________________________

____

Exercise A – Anatomy

1. Identify the major divisions of the autonomic nervous system shown in Figure 24-1.

    A. ______________________

    B. ______________________

    C. ______________________

    D. ______________________

    E. ______________________

    F. ______________________

    G. ______________________

    H. ______________________

    I. ______________________

    J. ______________________

    K. ______________________

2. Identify the structures of the external surface of the brain shown in Figure 24-2.

    A. ______________________

    B. ______________________

    C. ______________________

    D. ______________________

    E. ______________________

    F. ______________________

    G. ______________________

    H. ______________________

    I. ______________________

    J. ______________________

    K. ______________________

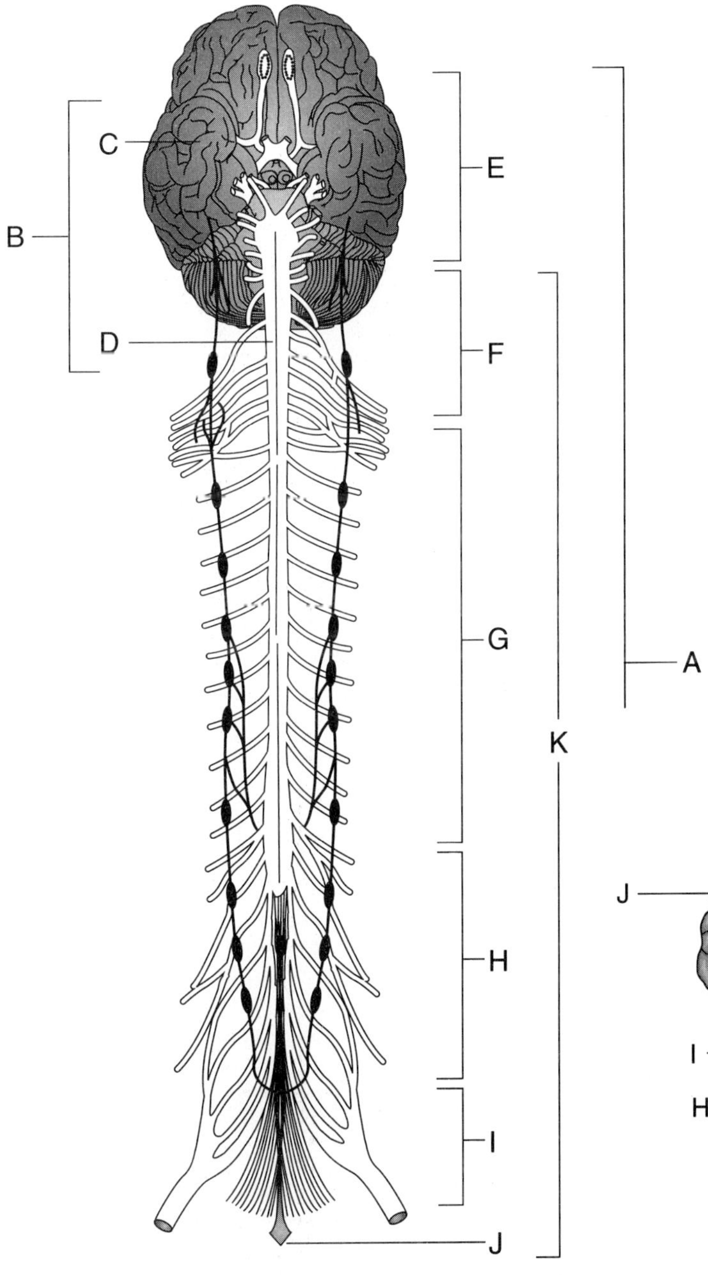

Figure 24-1

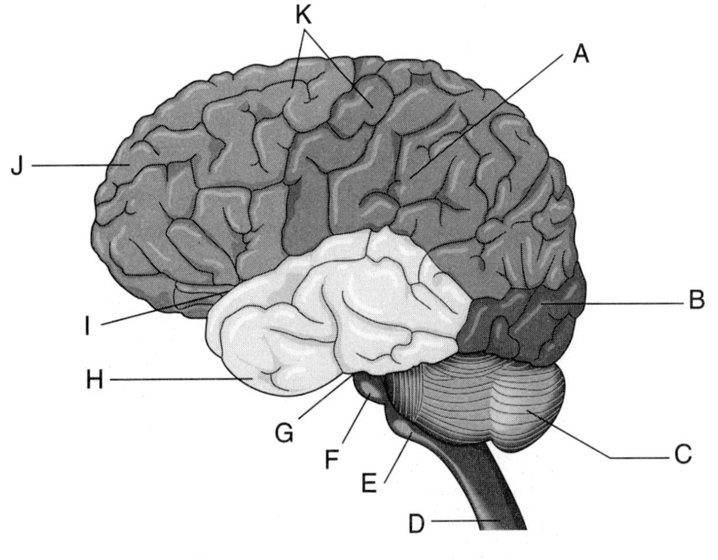

Figure 24-2

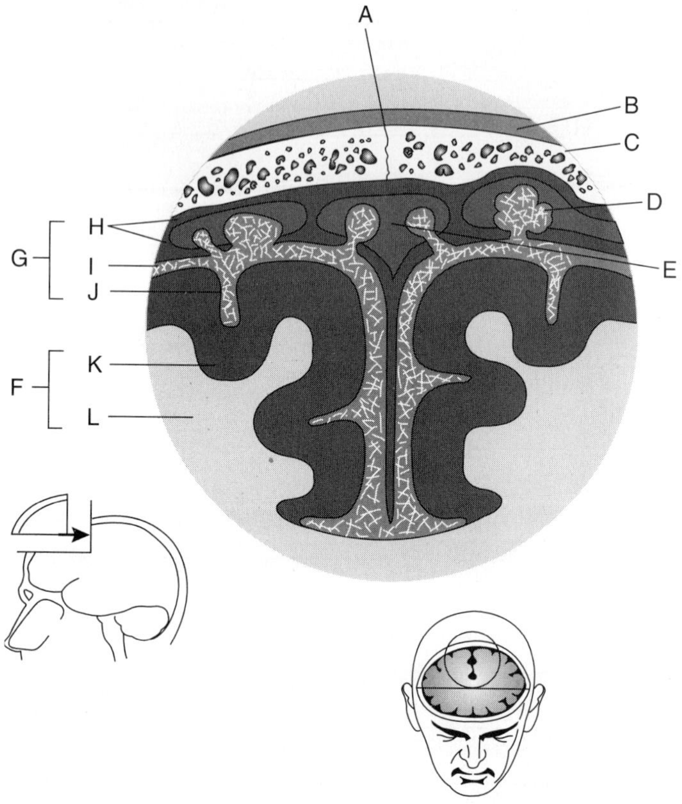

Figure 24-3

4. Identify the cranial nerves shown in Figure 24-4.

A. ____

B. ____

C. ____

D. ____

E. ____

F. ____

G. ____

H. ____

I. ____

J. ____

K. ____

L. ____

M. ____

3. Identify the meninges and related structures shown in Figure 24-3.

A. ____

B. ____

C. ____

D. ____

E. ____

F. ____

G. ____

H. ____

I. ____

J. ____

K. ____

L. ____

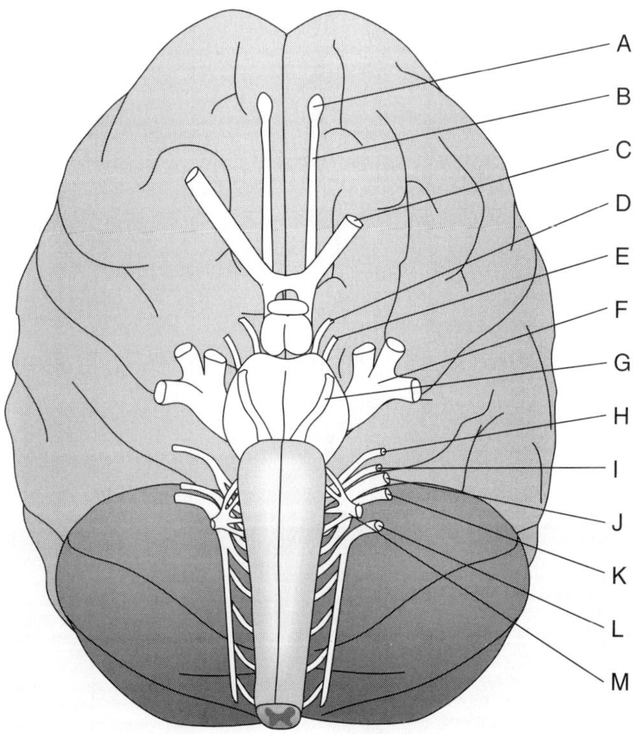

Figure 24-4

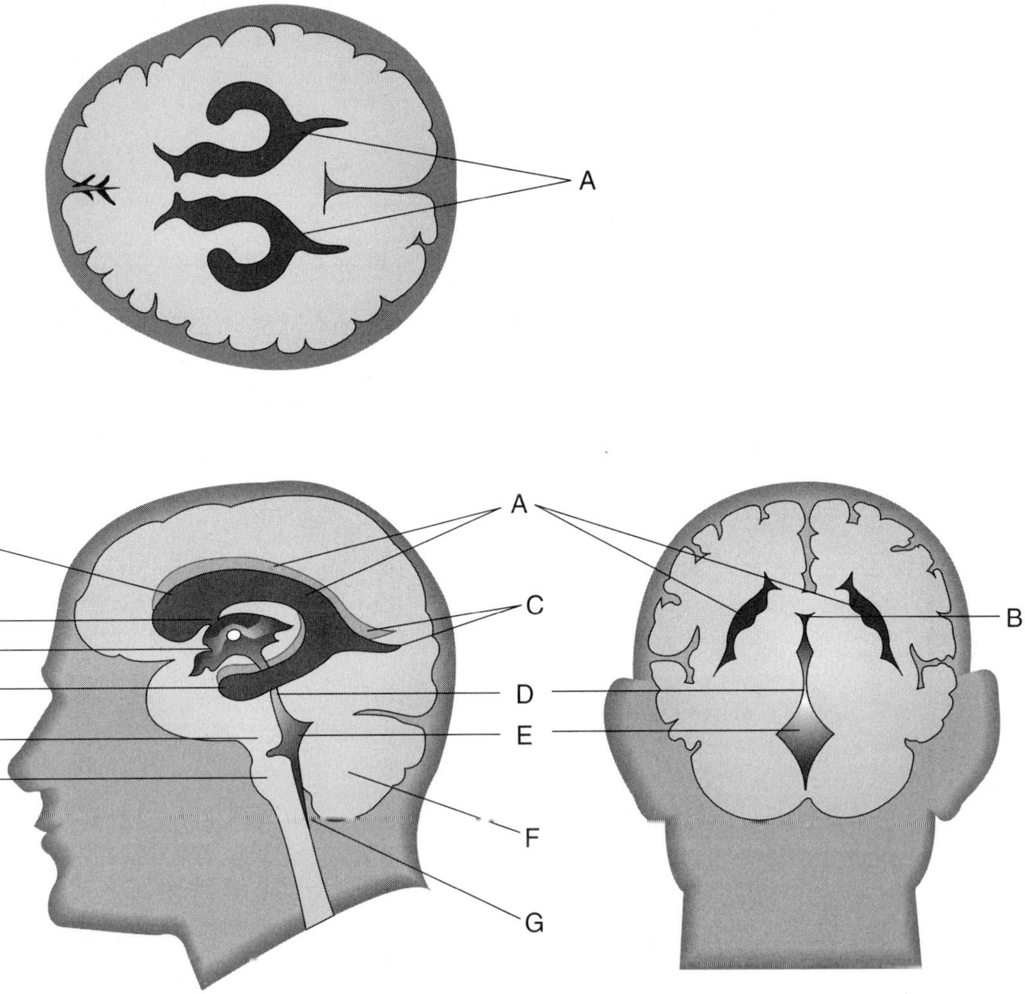

Figure 24-5

5. Identify the ventricles of the brain and related structures shown in Figure 24-5.

   A. ____________________

   B. ____________________

   C. ____________________

   D. ____________________

   E. ____________________

   F. ____________________

   G. ____________________

   H. ____________________

   I. ____________________

   J. ____________________

   K. ____________________

   L. ____________________

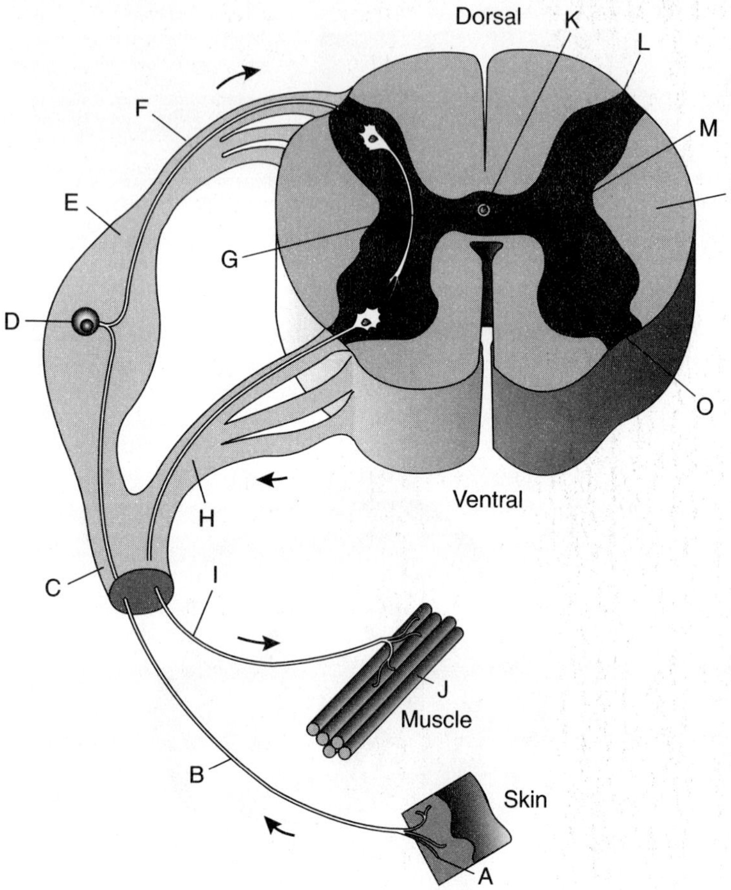

Figure 24-6

6. Identify the pathway of impulses (reflex arc) and related structures shown in Figure 24-6.

   A. ____________________

   B. ____________________

   C. ____________________

   D. ____________________

   E. ____________________

   F. ____________________

   G. ____________________

   H. ____________________

   I. ____________________

   J. ____________________

   K. ____________________

   L. ____________________

   M. ____________________

   N. ____________________

   O. ____________________

7. Name the eight bones of the cranium.

   A. ____________________

   B. ____________________

   C. ____________________

   D. ____________________

   E. ____________________

   F. ____________________

   G. ____________________

   H. ____________________

8. Name the three meningeal layers in sequence from outermost to innermost.

   A. ____________________

   B. ____________________

   C. ____________________

9. Where is CSF formed? How is it formed? __________

____

____

____

____

10. Name the three branches of the trigeminal nerve, and describe the functions of the target tissue(s) innervated by each branch.

A. ____________________________

____

B. ____________________________

____

C. ____________________________

____

11. What are the three primary functions of the nervous system?

A. ____________________________

____

B. ____________________________

____

C. ____________________________

____

12. What are the two subdivisions of the ANS, and what is the basic function of each division?

A. ____________________________

____

B. ____________________________

____

13. What is the circle of Willis? ____________

____

____

____

____

14. The auditory processing area of the brain is located in the ____________ lobe of the brain.

15. The vital centers of the brain (respiratory, cardiac, vasomotor) are contained in which portion of the brain stem? ____________________

____

____

____

____

Exercise B – Pathology

1. Hydrocephalus has several causes. List three.

A. ____________________________

B. ____________________________

C. ____________________________

2. List three types of obstruction of the aqueducts between the ventricles that can lead to hydrocephalus.

A. ____________________________

B. ____________________________

C. ____________________________

3. Describe the condition known as spondylosis.

____

____

____

____

____

4. Name two radiographic techniques that may be used to identify spinal disorders, and describe how each is used.

A. ____________________________

____

B. ____________________________

____

5. What is the difference between a subdural hematoma and an epidural hematoma? ____________________

____

____

____

____

6. Define craniosynostosis, and describe the method(s) for diagnosing the condition. ____________________

____

____

____

____

7. Describe spina bifida. ____________________

____

____

____

____

8. List the three classifications (locations) of spinal cord tumors and the symptoms of each.

A. ____________________

____

B. ____________________

____

C. ____________________

____

9. Carpal tunnel syndrome affects which nerve at what level? ____________________

____

____

____

____

10. What is the underlying cause of growth hormone (GH) overproduction? ____________________

____

____

____

____

11. Describe two symptoms that a patient with herniated nucleus pulposus may experience.

A. ____________________

B. ____________________

12. What is the most common type of brain tumor?

____

____

____

____

13. What symptoms are associated with acoustic neuroma? Which nerve is affected? ____________________

____

____

____

14. The condition known as tic douloureux is also known as ____________ ____________. What surgical procedure is performed to relieve the symptoms of tic douloureux? ____________________

____

____

____

15. List and describe the three types of subdural hematoma.

A. ____________________

____

B. ____________________

____

C. ____________________

____

Exercise C – Operation

1. What is the Mayfield pin-fixation device used to accomplish? ______________________________

2. How do Raney clips differ from aneurysm clips?

____

3. Access to the occipital lobe of the brain may be accomplished with the patient in either of two positions. Name the two possible positions.

   A. ______________________________

   B. ______________________________

4. What supplies may be necessary to remove scalp hair in the operating room? ______________________________

5. List three options for treatment of a cerebral aneurysm.

   A. ______________________________

   B. ______________________________

   C. ______________________________

6. It is important to restrict movement in and around the sterile field at all times, but why is this especially true during procedures near the cerebellopontine angle?

____

7. List the four main components of the ventriculoperitoneal shunt.

   A. ______________________________

   B. ______________________________

   C. ______________________________

   D. ______________________________

8. Name two approaches that can be used for surgery of the pituitary.

   A. ______________________________

   B. ______________________________

9. List two materials that can be implanted during cranioplasty and that can be molded to fit the cranial defect.

   A. ______________________________

   B. ______________________________

10. List two methods by which the bone flap is secured to the cranium following a craniotomy.

    A. ______________________________

    B. ______________________________

11. Why are two separate Mayo stands needed for transphenoidal procedures? ______________________________

12. What is papaverine used for during arterial intracranial surgery? ______________________________

13. What is the ideal temperature for irrigation fluid that will be used intracranially? ______________________________

14. What is the CUSA, and how is it used?

15. What is ICP? How is it monitored?

Exercise D – Specific Variations

Student Name ______________________ Date ____________

Instructor ______________________

Surgical Procedure – Student Case Study Report

The student will be provided with basic patient information (real or simulated) and is expected to complete the following case study.

1. Procedure name: ______________________
2. Definition of procedure: ______________________
3. What is the purpose of the procedure? ______________________
4. What is the expected outcome of the procedure?
5. Patient age: ______________________
6. Gender: ______________________
7. Additional pertinent patient information: ______________________
8. Probable preoperative diagnosis: ______________________
9. How was the diagnosis determined? ______________________
10. Discuss the relevant anatomy. ______________________
11. List the general and procedure-specific equipment that will be needed for the procedure.

12. List the general and procedure-specific instruments that will be needed for the procedure.

13. List the basic and procedure-specific supplies that will be needed for the procedure.

Pack

Basin

Gloves

Blades

Drapes

Drains

Dressings

Suture—Type of Suture, Needle (if applicable), and Anticipated Tissue Usage

Pharmaceuticals

Miscellaneous

14. Operative preparation:

15. What type of anesthesia will likely be used? Why?

16. List any special anesthesia equipment that may be needed.

17. Patient position during the procedure:

18. What supplies will be necessary for positioning?

____

____

____

____

19. What type of shave/skin preparation will be necessary (if any)? _______________

____

____

____

____

20. Define the anatomic perimeters of the prep.

____

____

____

____

21. List the order in which the drapes will be applied, and describe any specific variations.

____

____

____

____

____

____

____

22. List any practical considerations.

____

____

____

____

____

____

____

23. List the procedural steps, and describe the preparatory and supportive actions of the STSR during each step (use additional space if necessary).

Operative Procedure	Technical Considerations
1.	•
	•
2.	•
	•
3.	•
	•
4.	•
	•
5.	•
	•

(continues)

Operative Procedure *(continued)*	Technical Considerations *(continued)*
6.	•
	•
7.	•
	•
8.	•
	•
9.	•
	•
10.	•
	•

24. What is the postoperative diagnosis? ______________

25. Describe the immediate postoperative care.

26. What is the patient's long-term prognosis?

27. What are the possible complications? ______________

28. Comments or questions: ______________

29. What is the most valuable information you obtained from preparing this surgical procedure case study?

Case Studies

☐ CASE STUDY 1

Dr. Roberts was summoned to the emergency department to see a 34-year-old male who was brought in complaining of a severe headache of sudden onset. The patient described the headache as "violent, bursting, and explosive." He stated that it was the worst headache that he has ever experienced. The patient is nauseous, photophobic, and complaining of pain in the lower back. A lumbar puncture revealed blood within the cerebrospinal fluid.

1. What is the preliminary diagnosis? ______________________________

____

____

____

____

2. In addition to the lumbar puncture, what other diagnostic tests should be performed? ______________________________

____

____

____

____

3. What diagnostic test is considered the gold standard for this condition? ______________________________

____

____

____

____

4. What are the treatment options? ______________________________

____

____

____

____

☐

☐ CASE STUDY 2

Jamma, a 43-year-old secretary for a law firm, presents to Dr. Michaels with complaints of numbness, tingling, and pain in the right hand. Dr. Michaels notes during the examination that the symptoms are localized to the thumb, index finger, long finger, and medial aspect of the ring finger. He also notes that pain occasionally radiates up the arm into the shoulder. Jamma states that the pain awakens her at night.

1. What is the diagnosis? ________________________________

2. What is the etiology of the syndrome? ________________________________

3. How is the condition treated? List the conservative and surgical options. ________________________________

☐

Notes

Notes

Notes

Notes